Good Housekeeping

Family
First Aid

REVISED EDITION

Good Housekeeping

Family
First Aid

REVISED EDITION

MEDICAL EDITOR
Andy Jagoda MD, FACEP
Professor of Emergency Medicine
Mount Sinai School of Medicine
New York, New York

Contributing Editors

PETER SHEARER, MD
Assistant Professor
Mount Sinai School of Medicine
New York, New York

JESSICA FREEDMAN, MD
Assistant Professor
Mount Sinai School of Medicine
New York, New York

INTRODUCTION BY
SENATOR BILL FRIST, MD

Illustrated by David Kiphuth

A CMD PUBLISHING BOOK

HEARST BOOKS
A Division of Sterling Publishing Co., Inc.
NEW YORK

For Good Housekeeping
Editor in Chief: Ellen Levine
Special Projects Director: Richard Eisenberg

For CMD Publishing
Sarah Butterworth, Donna Balopole, Stacey Sharaby, Lynda Cranston, Linda Fetters,
Paul Perlow Design, Hermitage Publishing Services

The first aid procedures included in this book, if followed carefully, will help you
to deal with a wide range of emergencies. Whenever possible, however, you should
seek the services of professional medical personnel. The procedures described in
this book reflect the standard of knowledge and the accepted emergency practices
in the United States at the time of publication. You should stay informed of
changes in emergency care procedures, and it is also recommended that you take
a formal first aid and CPR training course.

Revised Edition 2004
Published by Hearst Books
A Division of Sterling Publishing Co., Inc.
387 Park Avenue South, New York, NY 10016

Good Housekeeping and Hearst Books are trademarks owned
by Hearst Communications, Inc.

Publisher's Note: Throughout this book, the pronouns "he" and "his" are often used to
refer to both sexes, except where a topic applies specifically to a man or a woman.

Library of Congress Cataloging-in-Publication Data
The Good housekeeping family first aid book / medical editor, Andy Jagoda ; contributing
editors, Peter Shearer, Jessica Freedman ; introduction by Bill Frist ; illustrated by David
Kiphuth.—2nd ed. p.cm.
    "A CMD Publishing book."
ISBN 1-58816-299-0
1. First aid in illness and injury—Popular works. I. Title: Family First Aid. II. Jagoda,
Andy. III. Shearer, Peter, M.D. IV. Freedman, Jessica. V. Good housekeeping.
RC87.G63 2004
616.02'52—dc22
2003057021

Printed in China

4 5 6 7 8 9 10

www.goodhousekeeping.com

For information about custom editions, special sales, premium and corporate
purchases, please contact Sterling Special Sales Department at 800-805-5489
or specialsales@sterlingpub.com.

Sterling ISBN-13: 978-1-58816-299-1
        ISBN-10: 1-58816-299-0

FOREWORD

If they offered a college degree in First Aid, I might well be a candidate for one, considering all the family emergencies I've dealt with as the mother of two sons. When the boys were young, it seemed as though we were constantly on the way to the doctor's office for some type of emergency. For example, my baby Danny's first steps toppled him, head first, into his toy chest, resulting in a cracked lip and lots of bleeding. Later, when I was in labor with my second son, Peter, Danny, then almost 4, had a 105° temperature. I was having contractions and Danny was hallucinating—that meant dunking my sick older child into a tepid bath at the same time I was getting ready to go to the labor room. Then there was the birthday party when one of the children fell into a rosebush in the garden, and we rushed her to the emergency room to have her scratched cornea treated. Whether the emergency involved rug burns from one of my sons being dragged across a carpet during roughhousing with his brother or knee-to-ankle abrasions from daring bicycle feats gone wrong, I learned to grit my teeth, hide my horror and fear, and just deal with it.

Surely my experiences are not so different from those most parents have. None of us is immune to medical crises; fortunately, most are handled well and effectively. Nevertheless, some emergencies require that we act immediately and methodically. And most arouse considerable anxiety and uncertainty.

That's why *The Good Housekeeping Family First Aid Book* is so valuable— at home, at work, in the car, on vacation. Through its wealth of detailed, easy-to-follow instructions, this book offers both guidance and comfort. The front of the book features a section on first aid basics—not only the ABC's of CPR, for example, but how to judge when someone is in distress and when to step in to help. Next, you'll find an A to Z listing of first aid topics— an alphabetical directory of specific emergencies describing what to look for and what to do (and what not to do). And since the best first aid strategy is to avoid accidents altogether, we've included a large section on prevention near the end of the book, and added a new section on safety preparation in today's turbulent world. In addition, we've put together a comprehensive resource section with phone numbers, Web sites, and addresses of first aid courses and helpful groups. Along the way, you'll see useful illustrations, handy sidebars, and prevention pointers.

The Good Housekeeping Family First Aid Book is an important manual that you can refer to often. Because, when you think about it, you too probably had the kind of life experiences to qualify for a degree in First Aid. But of course, what we really want is not a degree, but for our loved ones to stay safe, healthy, and strong so they'll survive life's inevitable bumps and bruises.

Ellen Levine
Editor in Chief
Good Housekeeping

The world changed dramatically on September 11, 2001, when the need for emergency preparedness and response suddenly became part of everyday life. The events of that day underscored the importance of each individual knowing how to respond quickly and efficiently to emergencies. Like the first edition, this revised edition of *The Good Housekeeping Family First Aid Book* is designed to assist the reader in preparing and responding to emergencies both large and small. I have worked carefully with Drs. Freedman and Shearer to update this home reference to meet the variety of first aid challenges potentially encountered in today's world. Thus, the sad realities of world events prompted the addition of an important new section on terrorism. It is my wish that the events of September 11th never be repeated, but I feel strongly that it is also my duty to prepare readers with the appropriate measures to take should tragedy strike.

Finding yourself in an emergency situation and not knowing what to do can be frightening. But by preparing for emergencies in advance, you can be in control during these events, act with confidence, and ultimately help save lives.

First aid has four essential components: prevention, preparation, recognizing an emergency, and using your resources. All four of these areas are described in *The Good Housekeeping Family First Aid Book*, in a clear, easy-to-follow presentation, designed to encourage and teach you both emergency prevention and action.

Prevention is a cornerstone to first aid. Whether you're at home or away from home, it's essential to think about prevention and to practice methods that can reduce the likelihood of an emergency occurring. For example, it's important to know how to splint a broken leg, but it's even better to prevent a fall in the first place by placing a no-skid mat underneath throw rugs! The Playing It Safe section shows you how to create a safer and healthier environment at home and away from home. Its pages are packed with preventive strategies, such as using life vests on boats, helmets for cycling, and childproof locks on cabinets; also included is a room-by-room checklist for the high-risk spots in your house.

Preparing for an emergency is key to responding effectively when an emergency strikes. Buying this book is a good first step. To prepare to administer first aid, you should also read the section Applying First Aid before an emergency occurs; take first aid courses; and maintain a well-stocked first aid kit. It's also a good idea to practice first aid skills on a regular basis and keep up to date with the latest first aid devices, such as automated external defibrillators.

Using your first aid skills well requires *knowing how to recognize an emergency* and then acting decisively and with confidence, with the best equipment available. Consequently, in designing the A to Z section of this book, care has been given not only to provide you with step-by-step descriptions of how to handle emergencies, but also to list signs and symptoms that can help you recognize what emergency event has occurred. Heart attack and stroke, for example, remain major causes of death and disability, yet both may be treated effectively if swift action is taken. Though you may not always be able to provide specific interventions to a victim of these emergencies, by recognizing their symptoms and acting quickly to obtain medical care you may help a victim survive.

Using your resources: Knowing how and where to go for help is the fourth component in providing first aid. Books are invaluable resources for preventing and handling emergencies. Moreover, information sources that are readily available, such as poison control centers, are especially valuable in helping you make important decisions. Many government and medical groups provide consumer information, and you can easily contact most of them through the Internet, where an explosion of medical information has taken place. To help you reach some of the best medical sites, the Resources section provides an annotated listing of more than 50 organizations, including addresses, phone numbers, and Web sites.

The goal of *The Good Housekeeping Family First Aid Book* is to stimulate and encourage you to think about preventing injuries and to guide you in recognizing emergencies and providing first aid. While many scenarios are described, it is not possible to discuss every possible situation that may occur. But the book provides you with a clear, basic approach that can be used to handle many emergencies, including what to do in a major crisis while you await professional medical care.

Andy Jagoda, MD
New York, New York

INTRODUCTION

Dear Readers,

The events of September 11th, and the anthrax attacks that followed, profoundly changed the way we think of safety—not only at our office buildings and airports, but in our homes, schools, post offices, and even at the shopping mall. We now know that there exist individuals and groups who seek to inflict bioterrorism against our free and open populace. Small amounts of deadly bacteria, viruses, or toxins released into the air, food or water supply, have the potential to threaten the lives of millions. As I wrote in my own book on family safety, *When Every Moment Counts*, bioterroism is no longer a question of if, but when, where and how.

I am gratified that the new edition of *The Good Housekeeping Family First Aid Book*, in addition to crucial information on family health and safety, includes information on biological and chemical threats. We've all been affected by this new reality. My wife, Karyn, and our three boys, Bryan, Jonathan, and Harrison, watched me live through the uncertainty of the anthrax attacks on the Capitol. I received many anxious questions from concerned parents regarding what they could do to protect their families. As I told them then, there is no reason for panic or paralysis in our everyday lives. There is good reason, however, for every American, young and old, to know much more about the threats that are emerging in these new and dangerous times. There are steps each of us can take to reduce our vulnerabilities and increase our security.

Every family should have a disaster plan. If your family does not have a disaster plan, start discussing one tonight at the dinner table. There are simple things you can do right away, like storing extra water, canned foods, batteries, and a change of clothes. We know, for example, from the blackout that enveloped major parts of the Northeast and Midwest in the summer of 2003 that every family should have a battery-operated radio.

The American Red Cross advises that your family's disaster plan should cover three essential elements:

Communication: How will you communicate with members in case of an emergency?
Destination: Where will family go if there is an attack?
Supplies: What supplies will you have on hand in case you need to "shelter at home" for a period of time?

This book will help you answer each of these questions and develop a plan that best addresses your family's needs and circumstances. As a physician, a father, and as the United States Senate Majority Leader, I urge you to take steps to protect your loved ones. Having this book on your shelf is an important start. Taking its instructions to heart will make a world of difference for you, your family, and for all of us who are in this together.

Sincerely,

Bill Frist, M.D.

CONTENTS

APPLYING FIRST AID

BEING PREPARED

You can never predict when an emergency will arise, so your best strategy is to be prepared. With preparation, you can act quickly, confidently, and in the proper manner, whatever the circumstances.

Having the right information and equipment at your fingertips is a good start.

•Post all telephone numbers of the doctor, emergency medical services (EMS—usually 911), local poison control center, and police and fire departments near the phone in your home or any other place that you and your family regularly visit. It's vital to have these numbers on hand in an obvious location. Dialing "0" in an emergency is not always a good choice, as the operator may be unfamiliar with your area and may not know how to reach your local EMS.

•Make sure your entire family knows where the emergency numbers are and how to dial them. It's a good idea to have your children practice calling (while you hold the receiver button down!), so they become familiar with the procedure.

•Note your own telephone number and address for your children, babysitters, or people staying at your home, so they can inform EMS or others in the event of an emergency.

•Keep your first aid kit up to date (see page 2) and ensure that all the members of your family, including the children, are familiar with the contents and know how and when to use them.

•Regularly check the status of your smoke and carbon monoxide (CO) detectors. Store all fire extinguishers in an accessible place and make sure the whole family knows where they are. Establish a fire escape plan and practice it at least twice a year.

HOME FIRST AID KIT

A well-stocked, well-organized first aid kit will help you respond effectively to medical emergencies around your home. The items that are listed below will provide you with the dressings and equipment you will need in most situations occurring in and around your home.

CONTENTS OF KIT

BANDAGES AND OTHER DRESSINGS
- Adhesive bandages of several sizes
- Adhesive tape
- Butterfly bandages
- Elastic roller bandages
- Triangular bandage (for a sling)
- Sterile gauze rolls and pads
- Sterile eye patches
- Sterile cotton balls

OTHER TOOLS
- Disposable sterile gloves or rubber gloves
- Safety pins
- Clean cloths and tissues
- Tweezers
- Sharp scissors with rounded tips
- Disposable, instant-activating cold packs
- Paper cups
- Bulb syringe
- Paper and pen/pencil
- Candle and matches
- Disposable face mask for mouth-to-mouth resuscitation
- Medicine spoon

MEDICATIONS
- Epinephrine auto-injector kit (such as EpiPen, EpiPen Jr.) if a family member has an allergy to bee stings, wasp stings, peanuts, or other substances
- Acetaminophen, ibuprofen, and aspirin—remember, aspirin should be given only to adults
- Syrup of ipecac—induces vomiting but should *only* be used on the advice of a doctor or poison control center
- Activated charcoal—used to inactivate poisons; may solidify in storage (check with package instructions or with manufacturer regarding storage guidelines)
- Diphenhydramine (Benadryl)
- Antacids (such as Mylanta)
- Antibiotic cream
- Calamine lotion

RESOURCES
- A copy of this book:
The Good Housekeeping Family First Aid Book
- List of emergency telephone numbers—doctor, emergency medical services (EMS), local poison control center, and police and fire departments. (Be sure to post these numbers by your telephone as well.)

TIPS FOR ASSEMBLY AND MAINTENANCE
- Choose the right container for your first aid kit. Look for a box that is lightweight, sturdy, waterproof, and dust proof. It should have a handle and a top that will shut securely. A plastic toolbox or fishing tackle box are good choices. Be sure to mark the container clearly as your home first aid kit.
- Keep your first aid kit in a cool, dry place (bathrooms are not always the best place for storage, as these rooms can be hot and humid). It should be stored well away from children and pets but be accessible enough so that you and other family members can reach it quickly.
- Check your first aid kit regularly, and replace any items that have been used. Discard any items with dates that have expired or are no longer sterile.
- Everyone (including all adults and responsible older children) should know the location and contents of your first aid kit. Go through the contents together and check that each person knows when and how to use them.

Take First Aid Training

Knowing how to take quick, effective action in an emergency can save lives. This book provides you with the first aid basics, but for truly comprehensive, hands-on training, there is no substitute for a first aid course including a basic life support (BLS) course from organizations such as the American Red Cross or National Safety Council or from other local groups in your area. Remember, it's better to know how to give first aid and never have to use it than to encounter an emergency situation and not know what to do. You should also be recertified in BLS on a regular basis.

FOR FURTHER INFORMATION...
See page 237 for information on where to find first aid courses.

WHEN IS IT AN EMERGENCY?

Recognizing an emergency is the first step in any first aid situation. Sometimes the seriousness of the situation is obvious, as in a motor vehicle accident or drowning. At other times, an emergency can be more subtle. But by understanding the nature of emergencies and becoming familiar with their signs, you can learn to recognize them in most cases. If you're ever in doubt, respond as though the situation is an emergency.

In general, an emergency involves an illness or injury that is life-threatening or that may cause severe or permanent damage to the victim. Listed below are signs of major illnesses or injuries that indicate an emergency exists.

Minor illnesses and injuries can usually be treated at home or by a doctor. Call your doctor if you're unsure what to do about minor medical situations.

Recognizing Major Injuries

Most major injuries are caused by sudden accidents such as bicycle, motorcycle, or car crashes, as well as choking, burns, electrocutions, smoke inhalation, poisoning, or severe animal bites.

A major injury may by recognized by
•Large or deep wound or burn
•Severe facial, head, neck, or back injuries

•External bleeding that is severe or that won't stop
•Signs of internal bleeding—dark red blood mixed with the stool; bright red blood covering the stool; black or tarry stool; urine that is red, "cola," or smoky in appearance; vomit that looks like coffee grounds; or bleeding from the vagina
•Sudden, severe, or persistent pain
•Sudden, severe, or persistent headache
•Continuous severe vomiting or diarrhea
•Marked changes in behavior—withdrawn, aggressive, or confused
•Paralysis, numbness, tingling, or weakness
•Signs of shock (see page 146)
•Signs of choking (see page 67)
•Difficulty breathing
•Irregular or no pulse
•Seizures (many seizures don't require emergency care—see page 139)
•Unconsciousness

You should always consider poisoning to be an emergency, including an overdose of prescription or over-the-counter medication, even if the victim shows no symptoms.

Recognizing Major Illnesses

Illness can strike unexpectedly, as in a heart attack or stroke. It can also result from poor control or worsening of chronic conditions, such as diabetes, asthma, or high blood pressure. While many minor illnesses can be safely handled at home, watch for the following signs that may indicate a major illness requiring emergency medical care:
•Signs of internal bleeding—dark red blood mixed with the stool; bright red blood covering the stool; black or tarry stool; urine that is red, "cola," or smoky in appearance; vomit that looks like coffee grounds; or bleeding from the vagina
•Sudden, severe, or persistent pain
•Pressure, squeezing, heaviness, or pain in the chest, usually behind the breastbone

DID YOU KNOW...

Poisoning can be the result of an overdose of prescription or over-the-counter medications, even when no symptoms are present. See page 131.

•Pain that spreads to the shoulder, neck, lower jaw, down the arm or into the back

•Continuous fever higher than 103°F

•Sudden weakness or numbness in face or arm or leg on one side of body

•Sudden blurred or lost vision

•Difficulty speaking or loss of speech

•Sudden, severe, or persistent headache

•Painful abdomen

•Stiff neck with fever

•Marked changes in behavior—withdrawn, aggressive, or confused

•Shock (see page 146)

•Difficulty breathing

•Irregular or no pulse

•Seizures (many seizures don't require emergency care— see page 139)

•Unconsciousness

GETTING EMERGENCY HELP

If the situation appears to be an emergency (or if you're unsure), the next step is to get help and to begin providing first aid. Depending on the nature of the illness, injury, or other medical condition, you should call EMS or the local poison control center. It may be tempting to call someone familiar, such as a family member, friend, or neighbor, but always seek help from trained emergency medical personnel first—they are your best bet in an emergency.

Emergency Medical Services (EMS)

EMS systems are designed to provide rapid response to emergency situations, first aid action at the scene, and quick, safe transport to a medical facility. There are several types of EMS systems across the United States with varying levels of training, skills, and experience (see Differences Between EMS Systems, page 7). The type of EMS

WHEN YOU CALL 911 . . .

Many areas across the United States now use an improved 911 service for access to emergency services. The new system displays not only your telephone number, but your name and location as well. This connection is retained until the EMS communications center releases it, so that your location information remains displayed. This system helps EMS reach you more quickly.

Many EMS centers also have special equipment that enables people with speech or hearing disabilities to communicate with a keyboard and printed message.

team that responds to your call will depend on both the geographic area you live in and its population base.

All EMS personnel are trained in first aid. They can do the following:
•Handle medical emergencies
•Correctly move the victim without causing further injury
•Treat some injuries at the emergency scene
•Transport the victim to the hospital quickly
•Improve the victim's chances of survival and recovery

Call EMS first when you see the signs of a major illness or injury (see page 3), or you encounter an emergency situation such as drowning or emergency childbirth.

WHEN CALLING EMS, YOU SHOULD PROVIDE
•The victim's precise location—street address and relevant apartment number, building floor or room number, as well as the nearest large intersection or other nearby landmarks
•Your name and telephone number
•A description of the emergency (describe signs and symptoms, such as chest pain or difficulty breathing)
•The number of people injured

Don't hang up until you're told to do so. You might be given instructions to follow over the phone until the ambulance arrives.

Poison Control Centers

Poison control centers are a telephone information resource for the public and health professionals on how to handle poisoning emergencies. These centers are staffed with trained personnel, usually qualified nurses trained in toxicology (the scientific study of poisons) who have access to information on thousands of poisonous substances. Medical doctors and other consultants are also on call in the event that more specific expertise is required.

DIFFERENCES BETWEEN EMS SYSTEMS

EMS systems vary greatly from community to community—in structure, staffing, training, and level of care delivered.

STRUCTURE

The type of EMS system available to you will depend on where you live:

•*Volunteer, nonprofit organizations* are often found in rural areas or those with a small population base, although they can also be located in larger, urban centers. They may be affiliated with the local volunteer fire department. Daytime EMS team members leave their jobs or homes, travel to the local EMS station, and respond to the emergency. At night, a crew may be based at the station.

•*Fire department-based EMS systems* fulfill both fire and EMS functions. Most of these systems provide emergency response and transport and depend on other agencies for nonemergency services. In some communities, EMS may be part of the police department.

•*Third-service agencies* are owned and operated by the local government or may be contracted for service from a private company. They are based at their own separate EMS stations and are run independent of police and fire services. In some areas, these agencies may depend on other agencies for first response and backup.

•*Hospital-based services* are usually managed as part of hospital departments and operate with significant input from hospital-based physicians. They provide nonemergency transport as well as local emergency response.

•*Private for-profit agencies* operate with limited financial support from the government and provide both emergency and nonemergency services.

STAFF AND TRAINING

Training and retraining requirements for EMS personnel differ widely from state to state. In fact, there are more than 40 levels of certification for emergency medical technicians (EMTs) across the country. Fortunately, training and practice standards have been established for four levels:

•*First responders* (including fire fighters, police officers, park rangers, and ski patrollers) are trained in basic life support, such as checking vital signs, providing resuscitation, and controlling bleeding.

•*EMT-Basics* are trained to provide basic emergency assessment and care, such as automated defibrillation and assisting victims with the use of their prescription medication, such as asthma medication.

•*EMT-Intermediates* have additional skills in specific aspects of advanced life support, which may include intravenous therapy and, in some states, the use of certain prescription medications.

•*EMT-Paramedics* have extensive training that covers a wide range of advanced life support skills from monitoring and interpretation of heart function to intubation (inserting a tube into the trachea to assist breathing).

First responders arrive first at the scene and initiate care, while more highly trained EMTs generally arrive at the scene 5 to 10 minutes after the first responders. Many, though not all, communities operate on a two-tiered system, while in other communities, there may be three separate teams that respond to an emergency call. In some areas, first responders are also trained in advanced life support.

TRANSPORT

Transportation methods for EMS can vary greatly as well. Ambulances are most commonly used, although quick-response vehicles are employed in some communities. They are designed to get EMS personnel to the scene quickly to start care while an ambulance is on its way.

In remote communities or in urban areas with heavy traffic, helicopters may transport EMS. Depending on the terrain, boats, airplanes, and other modes of transportation are also used.

Call your local poison control center when there has been an accidental or intentional poisoning or drug overdose (see also page 131). However, if you observe signs of severe injury or illness (see page 3), *always* call EMS first.

You can treat many poisonings successfully at home with the help of a poison control center. In more serious situations, the center will refer you to a doctor or hospital and will call ahead with specific information to help with the victim's care.

WHEN CALLING YOUR LOCAL POISON CONTROL CENTER, YOU SHOULD PROVIDE
- Your name and telephone number
- The victim's name, age, approximate weight, and current condition
- The exact name of the poison that has been taken
- When and how much poison was taken

HOW TO APPLY FIRST AID

BASIC LIFE SUPPORT

There is no substitute for a first aid basic life support (BLS) course with regular recertification.

An emergency situation can be daunting, even frightening. That's why it is vital to take control of an emergency situation at the outset (see Taking Control, page 9). Only then can you properly assess the scene and victim and apply the appropriate first aid techniques.

Assess the Scene

Before you begin helping a victim, take a brief moment to take stock of the scene.

- Determine whether you need to call EMS or, if appropriate, the poison control center. (Ideally, have someone else call while you attend to the victim; see When Is It an Emergency, page 3.)
- Look around, checking for any possible hazards, such as electrical lines or spilled chemicals. Determine whether it is safe to proceed. If not, or if you're in any doubt, don't go any further. Wait for EMS to arrive.
- Try to figure out what has happened. If others are nearby, ask them. If not, look for telltale clues, such

---

TAKING CONTROL

•Calm yourself. Take a few deep breaths and try to clear your mind of anxious thoughts.

•Think before you act. An emergency requires quick action, but it's better to act methodically and do the right thing than to rush and make a mistake.

•If the victim is conscious, obtain his consent before you begin first aid. (For more details, see What You Should Know About Good Samaritan Laws, page 26). If you don't know the victim, introduce yourself and ask if you can help.

•Calm the victim. Explain what you are doing as you do it. Be reassuring, but also be direct. Don't offer false hope.

•If the victim has medication, help him take it.

•Always treat the most serious injuries first.

•Remain focused on how you can help, rather than on any disturbing aspects of the emergency.

•Always try to protect the victim's privacy. Remove only as much of the victim's clothing as necessary to expose the injury.

•Ask all unnecessary bystanders to leave. If the victim has family or friends, they may stay at the scene, but ask them to leave ample room for you to work.

---

as an empty medicine container, or signs and symptoms, such as burns to the mouth. Check if the victim is wearing a medical identification tag.

•Examine the scene for any other victims.

Assess the Victim

When you encounter a victim, your first priority is to treat life-threatening injuries that are affecting his airway, breathing, and circulation. These are known as the ABCs.

AIRWAY

For air to enter the victim's body, the airway connecting the nose and mouth to the lungs must be kept open.

BREATHING

The victim must breathe so that oxygen can reach the heart and keep it pumping.

CIRCULATION

The victim must have a pulse (heartbeat) and enough blood to be circulated through the body to enable all body parts to function properly.

There are three main signs that indicate if a victim needs resuscitation:

1. No breathing
2. No pulse
3. Unconsciousness

It is possible that an unconscious victim may not be breathing but still has a pulse. In this case, only rescue breaths (or mouth-to-mouth breathing) may be needed.

If the victim is unconscious, is not breathing, and has no pulse, cardiopulmonary resuscitation (CPR) is called for. There are important differences in giving CPR to adults and children over age 8 (see page 13), children (ages 1 to 8; see page 16) and infants (less than 1 year old; see page 19). The technique for each age group is outlined separately.

Check for spinal injury

A possible spinal injury will influence how you treat a victim. That's why you should always suspect a spinal injury, especially if the victim shows signs of altered mental state, has sustained a head injury, has fallen, or has been in a car crash. As a general rule, you should assume that an unconscious victim has a spinal injury. If the victim is awake, alert, and has no neck pain, the chances of a spinal injury are less. (See Spinal Injury, page 154.)

Check for other injuries

Expose any other injuries, removing only as much of the victim's clothing as you need to. If necessary, cut away the clothing. Control any bleeding by using direct pressure (see Bleeding—External, page 38).

Watch for vomiting

If the victim vomits, turn him onto his left side. This is called the recovery position (page 11). It will help prevent further vomiting and will allow fluids to drain from the victim's mouth. If the victim is vomiting and you suspect a spinal injury, carefully log-roll the victim onto his left side as follows:

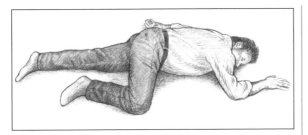

A victim who is vomiting should be placed in the recovery position.

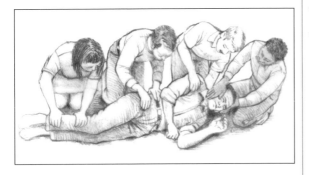

When a victim is vomiting and a spinal injury is suspected, carefully log-roll the victim onto his left side.

•Position yourself at the victim's head and keep his head and shoulders in a fixed position. Others should position themselves at the victim's side, supporting his waist and legs. Gently roll the victim as a unit toward the people supporting his body (waist and legs), always keeping his head in line with his body.

•If you're alone, hold the victim's neck steady just below the back of his head. *DO NOT* log-roll the victim until help arrives.

Prevent or reduce shock

If the victim is showing signs of shock (such as pale, cold, clammy skin; sweating; skin around the mouth and lips is blue; nausea and vomiting; rapid shallow breathing; fast pulse that may become weaker; anxiety; dizziness and lightheadedness—see page 146), place him in the shock position:

•Lay the victim down with legs elevated (to increase blood flow to the heart and brain).

•Cover the victim with blankets or coats to keep him warm.

To prevent or reduce shock, place the victim in the shock position, and then cover him with blankets or coats to keep him warm.

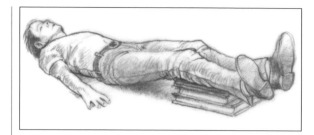

DO NOT use the shock position if
• The victim is having difficulty breathing
• You suspect a neck or other spinal injury
• The position makes him uncomfortable

CPR Techniques

CPR (cardiopulmonary resuscitation) is a combination of rescue breathing that supplies oxygen to the body and chest compressions that mimic the heart's job of pumping the oxygen-rich blood around the body.

WHAT NOT TO DO: PREVENTING FURTHER INJURY

In an emergency situation, your goal is to assess the victim and provide appropriate first aid. It's equally important to prevent further injury to the victim. How can you do that? By following these essential guidelines:
• *DO NOT* provide first aid if the victim refuses it.
• *DO NOT* attempt to transport a severely injured or ill victim to the hospital, unless there is no other way to obtain medical assistance.
• *DO NOT* attempt a first aid technique if you're not sure how to perform it. Wait for EMS instead.
• *DO NOT* block an unconscious victim's airway. If the victim is unconscious
  • *DO NOT* give him food or drink.
  • *DO NOT* place a pillow under his head.
  • *DO NOT* lay him on his back if he has vomited, unless you have to provide rescue breaths or CPR.
• *DO NOT* move a victim if you suspect a

spinal injury, unless absolutely necessary. (See Moving a Spinal Injury Victim, page 156).
• *DO NOT* be rough or shake a victim. Always use smooth, gentle motions.
• *DO NOT* hold a victim down if he is having a seizure.
• *DO NOT* induce vomiting by placing your fingers or another object down a victim's throat.
• *DO NOT* add to a victim's pain. If the victim finds any position or treatment uncomfortable, change or stop it immediately.
• *DO NOT* remove an impaled object (such as a knife). Stabilize the object in place with bulky dressings. Never apply direct pressure on an impaled object or protruding bone when attempting to control bleeding.
• *DO NOT* move an injured limb (like a broken bone or dislocation) without supporting and immobilizing it first.

The goal of CPR is to restore circulation. On its own, CPR will not always completely revive the victim, but it will "buy time," providing oxygen to the brain and heart until the EMS team arrives. CPR for adults and children over age 8, young children (ages 1–8), and infants (under 1 year) is outlined below. Be sure to use the right technique for the victim's age.

CPR FOR ADULTS AND CHILDREN OVER AGE 8

•Call 911 (EMS).
•Check if the victim is conscious. You can find out by calling the victim's name or gently tapping him on the shoulder.

IF THE VICTIM IS CONSCIOUS AND BREATHING

•Check his pulse by placing two fingers (but not your thumb) on the carotid artery located at the side of the neck. You can find this artery by placing your fingers on the victim's Adam's apple, then sliding the fingers into the groove of the neck on the side closest to you.
•A victim's condition can worsen at any time, so monitor his ABCs (as below) regularly and treat as necessary until EMS arrive.

IF THE VICTIM IS CONSCIOUS BUT IS HAVING DIFFICULTY BREATHING

•The victim may be choking. If this appears to be the case, perform the Heimlich maneuver (see Rescue Maneuvers, page 69).

IF THE VICTIM IS UNCONSCIOUS

•Position the victim on his back so you can check his ABCs. If the victim is lying on his side or stomach, you will have to turn him onto his back. If possible, have others help you do the following:
  •Carefully straighten his legs.
  •Use one hand to support his head and neck and then place your other hand on the far side of his body.

REMEMBER AED

Automated external defibrillators (AEDs) are small, easy-to-use devices that deliver an electric shock to the heart, restoring a normal heartbeat. More and more, AEDs are available in public places, such as airports. Whenever a victim is unconscious, not breathing, and has no pulse, an AED, together with CPR, can vastly improve his chances for survival. (See Automated External Defibrillators, page 21.)

MAKE PROTECTION A PRIORITY

Always bear in mind the risk of exposure to infection while giving CPR, particularly if you're helping someone you don't know. Using a disposable face mask for rescue breathing will protect you from a victim's saliva and possible infection. It will also protect the victim if you have an existing infection (for more details, see The Risk of Disease, page 25).

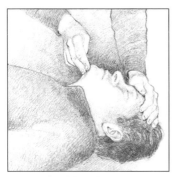

Opening the victim's airway.

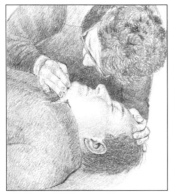

Checking the victim's breathing.

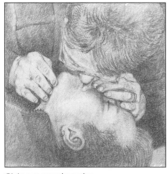

Giving rescue breaths.

•Log-roll the body in one smooth motion, always keeping the victim's head in line with his body.

•*DO NOT* rotate his head, neck, shoulders, or pelvis.

Airway

Open the victim's airway.

•Place yourself at right angles to the victim.

•Place one hand on the victim's forehead and gently push downward so the head tilts backward.

•Place the index and middle fingers of your other hand under the chin to lift the victim's jaw.

•If you suspect a spinal injury (see page 154), begin by lifting the chin only. If this doesn't open the airway, very gently tilt the head backward.

Breathing

Look, listen, and feel for the victim's breathing.

•*Look:* Is the victim's chest rising and falling?

•*Listen:* Place your ear next to the victim's nose and mouth. Can you hear his breaths?

•*Feel:* Put your cheek next to the victim's nose and mouth. Can you feel the breaths?

If the victim is not breathing, give rescue breaths

•Keep the victim's head back and chin tilted (as described above).

•Pinch the victim's nose shut.

•Take a deep breath.

•Place your mouth tightly over the victim's mouth.

•Give 2 slow rescue breaths, ensuring the victim's chest rises each time, then falls before giving another breath. Each breath should last $1^{1}/_{2}$ to 2 seconds.

If the victim is still not breathing, his airway is likely blocked. You must try to dislodge the object (see Rescue Maneuvers, page 69).

Circulation

•Feel for a pulse—place two fingers (but not your thumb) on the carotid artery located at the side of the neck. You can find this artery by placing your

CPR

fingers on the victim's Adam's apple, then sliding the fingers into the groove of the neck on the side closest to you. Use your other hand to keep the victim's head tilted.

•Look for and control any severe bleeding.

•Observe the victim's skin—poor or no circulation is indicated by clammy, cool, pale skin. Light-skinned people may appear blue or gray around the mouth and lips. In dark-skinned people, check the color of the nail beds or inside the mouth.

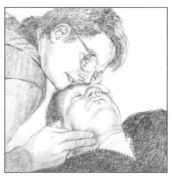

Checking for a pulse.

IF THERE IS NO CIRCULATION, START CHEST COMPRESSIONS COMBINED WITH RESCUE BREATHING

•Keep one hand on the victim's forehead to maintain the head tilt. With your other hand, locate the base of the breastbone at the center of the chest where the ribs form a **V**.

•With one hand, place your middle finger on the **V** and your index finger next to it. Place the heel of your other hand beside and above your index finger. Remove your fingers from the **V** and place the heel of this hand over the top of the other, intertwining your fingers.

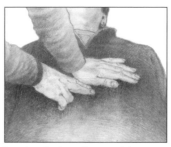

Locating the breastbone and the spot for chest compression.

•Position your shoulders directly over your hands by shifting your weight upward and forward. Your arms should be straight with elbows locked.

•Shifting your weight to your hands, compress the victim's chest by $1^{1}/_{2}$ to 2 inches. Be sure to push straight down. Do this 15 times at a rate of slightly over 1 compression per second (80 compressions per minute). Release between compressions by lifting up, but don't shift or remove your hands. Count out loud as you push to keep track.

•Provide 2 rescue breaths, followed by 15 compressions. Repeat this sequence for a total of 4 cycles (about 1 minute).

•Check the victim's breathing and pulse.

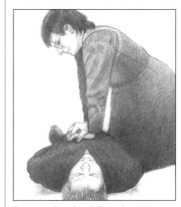

Compressing the victim's chest.

•If a pulse hasn't returned, resume CPR until EMS arrive or until you are too exhausted to continue.

•If a pulse has returned but breathing hasn't, stop compressions and continue rescue breathing.

CHILDREN AND CHOKING

When a child is having difficulty breathing, a blocked airway (choking), rather than a heart problem, is often the culprit. If a child appears to be choking, your *first* step is to begin resuscitation techniques (including the Heimlich maneuver) before you do anything else. Done properly, these techniques can often dislodge the foreign object, clear the child's airway, and restore his breathing (see also Choking, page 67).

•If breathing and pulse have returned, place the victim in the recovery position (see page 11) and monitor him until EMS arrive.

CPR FOR YOUNG CHILDREN (AGES 1–8)

•Check if the child is conscious. You can find out by calling the child's name or gently tapping him on the shoulder.

•Begin resuscitation techniques first (see below).

•Call 911 (EMS) if the child does not fully recover.

IF THE CHILD IS CONSCIOUS AND BREATHING

•Check his pulse by placing two fingers (but not your thumb) on the carotid artery located at the side of the neck. You can find this artery by placing your fingers on the child's Adam's apple and then sliding the fingers into the groove of the neck on the side closest to you.

•A victim's condition can worsen at any time, so regularly monitor his ABCs (as below) and treat as necessary until EMS arrive.

IF THE CHILD IS CONSCIOUS BUT IS HAVING DIFFICULTY BREATHING

•The child may be choking. If this appears to be the case, perform the Heimlich maneuver (see Rescue Maneuvers, page 69).

IF THE CHILD IS UNCONSCIOUS

•Position the child on his back so you can check his ABCs. If the child is lying on his side or front, you will have to turn him onto his back. If possible, have others help you do the following:

   •Carefully straighten his legs.

   •Use one hand to support his head and neck and place your other hand on the far side of his body.

   •Log-roll the body in one smooth motion, always keeping the child's head in line with the rest of his body.

   •*DO NOT* rotate his head, neck, shoulders, or pelvis.

Airway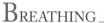

Open the child's airway:

•Place yourself at right angles to the child.

•Place one hand on the child's forehead and gently push downward so the head tilts backward.

•Place the index and middle fingers of your other hand under the chin to lift the child's jaw.

•If you suspect a spinal injury (see page 154), begin by lifting the chin only. If this doesn't open the airway, very gently tilt the head backward.

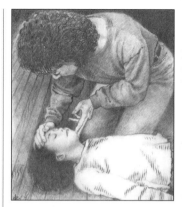

Opening the child's airway.

Breathing

Look, listen, and feel for breathing.

•*Look:* Is the child's chest rising and falling?

•*Listen:* Place your ear next to the child's nose and mouth. Can you hear his breaths?

•*Feel:* Put your cheek next to the child's nose and mouth. Can you feel the breaths?

IF THE CHILD IS NOT BREATHING, GIVE RESCUE BREATHS

•Keep the child's head back and chin tilted (as described above).

•Pinch the child's nose shut.

•Take a deep breath.

•Place your mouth tightly over the child's mouth.

•Give 2 slow rescue breaths, ensuring the child's chest rises each time, then falls before giving another breath. Each breath should last 1 to $1^{1}/_{2}$ seconds.

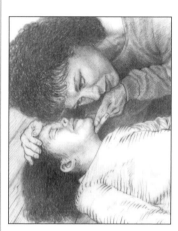

Checking the child's breathing.

If the child is still not breathing, his airway is likely blocked. You must try to dislodge the object (see Rescue Maneuvers, page 69).

Circulation

•Feel for a pulse—place two fingers (but not your thumb) on the carotid artery located at the side of the neck. You can find this artery by placing your fingers on the child's Adam's apple, then sliding the fingers into the groove of the neck on the side

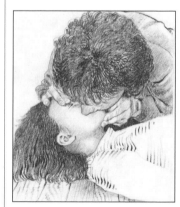

Giving rescue breaths.

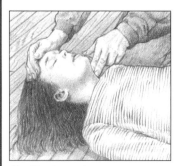

Checking for a pulse.

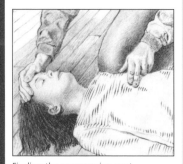

Finding the compression spot.

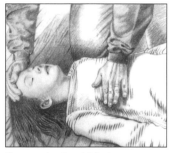

Compressing the child's chest.

closest to you. Use your other hand to keep the child's head tilted.

•Look for and control any severe bleeding.

•Observe the child's skin—poor or no circulation is indicated by clammy, cool, pale skin. Light-skinned children may appear blue or gray around the mouth and lips. In dark-skinned children, check the color of the nail beds or inside the mouth.

IF THERE IS NO CIRCULATION, START CHEST COMPRESSIONS COMBINED WITH RESCUE BREATHING

•Keep one hand on the victim's forehead to maintain the head tilt. With your other hand, locate the base of the breastbone at the center of the chest where the ribs form a **V**.

•With one hand, place your middle finger on the **V** and your index finger next to it. Notice the location of your index finger. Then lift the fingers and place the heel of this hand just above where your index finger was previously. Keep your fingers off the child's chest while you push.

•Compress the child's chest by 1 to $1^{1}/2$ inches. Be sure to push straight down. Give 5 compressions in about 3 seconds (a rate of about 100 compressions per minute). Release between compressions by lifting up, but don't shift or remove your hand. Count out loud as you push to keep track.

•Provide 1 rescue breath, followed by 5 compressions. Repeat this sequence for a total of 4 cycles (about 1 minute).

•Check the child's pulse and breathing.

  •If a pulse hasn't returned, resume CPR until EMS arrive or until you are too exhausted to continue.

  •If a pulse has returned but breathing hasn't, stop chest compressions and continue rescue breathing.

  •If breathing and pulse have returned, place the child in the recovery position (see page 11) and monitor the child until EMS arrive.

CPR FOR INFANTS (UNDER 1 YEAR)

•Check if the infant is conscious. You can find out by gently tapping him on the shoulder.

•Begin resuscitation techniques first (see below).

•Call 911 (EMS) if the infant does not fully recover.

IF THE INFANT IS CONSCIOUS AND BREATHING

•Check his pulse by placing two fingers (but not your thumb) on the brachial artery located on the inside of the upper arm, between the infant's elbow and armpit.

•A victim's condition can worsen at any time, so regularly monitor his ABCs (as below) and treat as necessary until EMS arrive.

IF THE INFANT IS CONSCIOUS BUT HAVING DIFFICULTY BREATHING

•The infant may be choking. If this appears to be the case, perform rescue maneuvers (see page 72).

IF THE INFANT IS UNCONSCIOUS

•Position the infant on his back so you can check his ABCs. If the infant is lying on his side or stomach, you will have to turn him onto his back by doing the following:

>•Carefully straighten his legs.

>•Use one hand to support his head and neck and place your other hand on the far side of his body.

>•Log-roll the body in one smooth motion, always keeping the infant's head in line with his body.

>•*DO NOT* rotate his head, neck, shoulders, or pelvis.

AIRWAY

Open the infant's airway.

•Place yourself at right angles to the infant.

•Place one hand on the infant's forehead and gently push downwards so the head tilts backward.

•Place the index finger of your other hand under the chin to lift the infant's jaw. *DO NOT* use your thumb.

•If you suspect a spinal injury (see page 154), begin

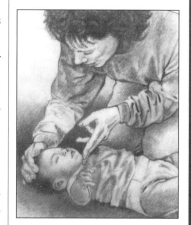

Opening the infant's airway.

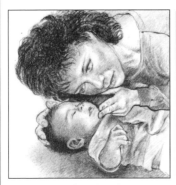

Checking the infant's breathing.

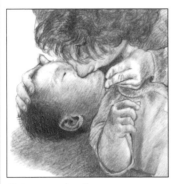

Giving rescue breaths.

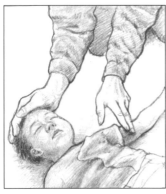

Checking the infant's pulse.

by lifting the chin only. If this doesn't open the airway, very gently tilt the head backward.

BREATHING

Look, listen, and feel for breathing.

•*Look:* Is the infant's chest rising and falling?

•*Listen:* Place your ear next to the infant's nose and mouth. Can you hear his breaths?

•*Feel:* Put your cheek next to the infant's nose and mouth? Can you feel the breaths?

IF THE INFANT IS NOT BREATHING, GIVE RESCUE BREATHS

•Keep the infant's head back and chin tilted (as described above).

•Take a deep breath.

•Place your mouth tightly over the infant's mouth and nose.

•Give 2 slow rescue breaths, making sure that the infant's chest rises each time, then falls before giving another breath. Each breath should last 1 to 1½ seconds.

If the infant is still not breathing, his airway is likely blocked. You must try to dislodge the object (see Rescue Maneuvers for Babies, page 72).

CIRCULATION

•Feel for a pulse—place two fingers (but not your thumb) on the brachial artery located on the inside of the upper arm, between the infant's elbow and armpit. Use your other hand to keep the infant's head tilted.

•Look for and control any severe bleeding.

•Observe the infant's skin—poor or no circulation is indicated by clammy, cool, pale skin. Light-skinned infants may appear blue or gray around the mouth and lips. In dark-skinned infants, check the color of the nail beds or inside the mouth.

IF THERE IS NO CIRCULATION, START CHEST COMPRESSIONS COMBINED WITH RESCUE BREATHING

•Keep one hand on the victim's forehead to maintain the head tilt.

•Imagine a line connecting the infant's nipples. Place three fingers on the breastbone with your index finger just below this imaginary line.

•Raise your index finger and use the other two fingers to give chest compressions. Be sure to push straight down.

•Compress the infant's chest by $1/2$ to 1 inch. Give 5 compressions in about 3 seconds (a rate of about 100 compressions per minute). Release between compressions by lifting up, but don't shift or remove your fingers. Count out loud as you push to keep track.

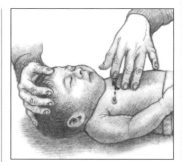

Locating the compression point and compressing the infant's chest.

•Provide 1 rescue breath, followed by 5 compressions. Repeat this sequence for a total of 4 cycles (about 1 minute).

•Check the infant's pulse and breathing.

•If a pulse hasn't returned, resume CPR until EMS arrive or until you are too exhausted to continue.

•If a pulse has returned but breathing hasn't, stop compressions and continue rescue breathing.

•If breathing and pulse have returned, place the infant in the recovery position (see page 11) and monitor him until EMS arrive.

Automated External Defibrillators

When a victim has no pulse, it means that his heart has ceased to pump blood around the body. This is called cardiac arrest. It often occurs when the heart experiences an electrical malfunction and begins to beat in an abnormal, chaotic manner (called ventricular fibrillation), causing the heart's pumping function to stop immediately.

The lifesaving technique of CPR (described above) restores some blood flow in a victim in cardiac arrest and buys important time until EMS arrive. But CPR, on its own, will not completely reverse cardiac arrest. The best way to accomplish that is with defibrillation. This technique provides an electric shock to the heart to restore a normal heartbeat.

Defibrillators (the devices used to provide the electric shock) have long been used by doctors in

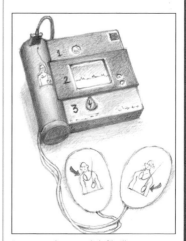

Automated external defibrillator

AED LAWS

Lay rescuers (the public)—with proper training—are being granted permission to use AEDs in an ever-increasing number of states. Check with your local EMS office or a lawyer regarding the law in your state.

AED CAUTIONS

AEDs are not for everyone and not for every situation. *DO NOT* use an AED in the following circumstances:

•The victim is in water or on a wet surface.
•The victim is lying on a metal surface.
•The victim is under 8 years of age or weighs less than 70 pounds.

If the victim is wearing a medication patch, don't place the AED pads directly on top of the patch. Remove the patch and clean the area first.

hospital settings or by trained emergency personnel at emergency scenes to save victims in cardiac arrest. Advances in computer technology have produced the automated external defibrillator (AED). This is a simpler, more compact version of the standard defibrillator. It can be used in a variety of settings and by a variety of people, although who is allowed to use an AED varies from state-to-state.

Increasingly, AEDs are being placed in public places such as stadiums, office buildings, and airplanes. This is good news considering that survival rates in cardiac arrest victims are dramatically improved with AEDs.

Operating and maintaining an AED is simple and straightforward, and in many states non-medical people can operate AEDs if they are properly trained. The Food and Drug Administration (FDA) has approved AEDs for home use, but only with a doctor's prescription and only if potential users have received appropriate training. This is usually reserved for families of people with severe heart disease. Check with a lawyer or your local EMS office to determine the law in your area regarding the home use of AEDs. Keep in mind that AEDs are not recommended for every household.

HOW TO USE AN AED

An AED, if available at the emergency scene, should be used in conjunction with CPR.

Be aware that there are several different models of AEDs and minor variations may exist in applying and using the device.

AT AN EMERGENCY SCENE

•If you are alone, call 911 (EMS) and get the AED (see AED Cautions).

•If someone is with you, tell him to call 911 (EMS) and to get the AED. Check the victim's ABCs. If he is unconscious, not breathing, and has no pulse, begin CPR. Continue CPR while the AED is being set up.

SETTING UP AND USING THE AED

•Place the AED near the victim's left ear.

•Open the AED and turn the power on.

•Remove the victim's clothing to expose his chest.

•Attach the electrode pads to the victim's chest—one to the right side of the breastbone between the nipple and collarbone, the other to the outside of the left nipple, just below the left armpit. A diagram on the packaging demonstrates the proper position of the pads. But, even if they are not in the exact position, the AED will work.

•"Clear" the victim (this means you should stop CPR and make sure no one is touching the victim).

•Press the analyze button. The AED will then analyze the victim's heart rhythm to determine whether a shock should be given.

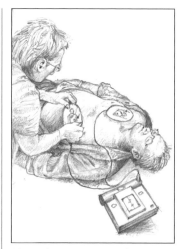

When using an AED, open the victim's shirt and place one pad between the nipple and collarbone and the other below the victim's left armpit.

IF A SHOCK **IS** INDICATED

•"Clear" the victim.

•Press the shock button.

•"Clear" the victim and analyze again.

•Repeat this up to 3 times, if shock is indicated.

•If still no pulse, start CPR.

IF **NO** SHOCK IS INDICATED

•Check the victim's pulse.

•If there is a pulse, check breathing.

•If no breathing, provide rescue breaths. If breathing, log-roll the victim onto his left side in the recovery position and monitor until EMS arrive.

•If no pulse, resume CPR for 1 minute and recheck. If there is still no pulse, begin AED steps again (as above).

The Heimlich Maneuver

The Heimlich maneuver is a simple, effective procedure that is used when a victim is choking. This thrusting technique rapidly forces air from the victim's lungs and dislodges the object blocking a victim's airway. The Heimlich maneuver involves abdominal thrusts. If the victim is large, either because of obesity or the later stages of pregnancy, or is under 1 year of age, chest thrusts are used instead; back blows are another rescue maneuver used in children under 1 year of age.

Choking is an all-too-common and life-threatening incident. By learning the Heimlich maneuver, chest thrusts, and back blows, you will be prepared and potentially save lives. For complete details on performing these maneuvers see Choking, page 67.

PRECAUTIONS AND GUIDELINES FOR THE RESCUER

Don't Become a Victim! Preventing Injury to the Rescuer

There are risks in any emergency situation. Risks to the victim may be obvious, but what about potential dangers to you, the rescuer? You need to be aware of your own well-being and use caution and common sense in an emergency. By doing so, you will not only be safeguarding yourself but also providing more effective help to the victim.

YOUR PHYSICAL CONDITION

Be honest with yourself. If you have a physical condition that could restrict your activity or movement, such as a bad back or a chronic condition such as angina, be aware of your limits and stay within them. Emergency situations are usually demanding, so be sure to listen to your body and heed its message.

YOUR EMOTIONAL STATE

As noted at the beginning of this chapter, there are some steps you can take to try and calm yourself at an emergency scene. But if you find that panic and anxiety are taking over, wait for EMS. To be an effective rescuer, you need to be in control of your emotions—and your actions.

DANGEROUS SCENES

Fire, downed electrical wires, ice water—these are just some of the dangerous situations you might encounter in and around your home. Before you attempt to help a victim in an unsafe environment, consider your own safety and always proceed cautiously. Assess the scene: If it appears unsafe in any way, or if you suspect danger, don't proceed. Call 911 (EMS) and wait for them to arrive. Remember, if you become injured, you can't help the victim, and you will become a victim yourself.

THE RISK OF DISEASE

Blood is a common element in many emergencies. As a rescuer, you may be exposed to a victim's blood, and the victim may be exposed to your blood as well. This can be a concern because some viral diseases, such as HIV (the virus that causes AIDs) and hepatitis B and C, can be spread through blood.

When providing first aid to a family member, relative, or friend, you will probably know whether he has a serious illness or infection. But, if you help a coworker or stranger, you can never be sure. Another consideration is your own health status. Do you have, or suspect you have, a serious illness or infection that could be transmitted through the blood?

The "better safe than sorry" adage applies to emergency situations. By taking the following precautions, you can reduce the risk of disease to yourself and the victim.

• Always wash your hands before and after providing first aid.

• If you have an open cut, cover it with an adhesive bandage.

• If the victim is bleeding, try to reduce contact with the blood by using sterile disposable gloves or any other clean, available barrier such as rubber gloves, cloths, dressings, or plastic wrap.

• Try to avoid contact with clothes or other objects soiled by blood or body fluids.

• *DO NOT* put your hands near your eyes, nose, or mouth while giving first aid.

• *DO NOT* eat or drink while giving first aid.

Seek immediate medical care if you are unsure about a victim's health status and have been exposed to his blood or body fluids.

When a victim needs rescue breathing, you will be exposed to his saliva. Most serious illnesses and infections are not passed through the saliva. Still, if you think you may be providing rescue breaths to a person you don't know well, you may consider purchasing disposable face masks and storing them in your first aid kit. These devices come in different sizes for use with adults, children, or infants and will protect you from a victim's saliva.

What You Should Know About Good Samaritan Laws

In some emergency situations, you might worry about providing first aid. What if something goes wrong? Will you be held responsible?

In most states, Good Samaritan laws have been enacted to provide legal protection to people who give first aid to ill or injured people. These laws were created to address concerns of would-be rescuers and to encourage them to help out in emergency situations.

Under the Good Samaritan laws, you are protected in most cases from being sued or found financially responsible if you act in good faith and in a responsible manner by following basic first aid guidelines:

•Calling either 911 (EMS) or the local emergency number

•Not moving a victim unless the situation is unsafe

•Asking a conscious victim for his permission before providing first aid

•Monitoring the victim and providing care until EMS arrive

•Not using first aid treatments that exceed your training or skill level

Good Samaritan laws assume that each person will do his best to save a victim's life or prevent further injury. In cases where a rescuer has been reckless or negligent, or has abandoned the scene (in other words, *not* done his best for the victim), the court ruled that protection of these laws did not apply. Rest assured, however, that this is uncommon, and people are rarely sued for helping in an emergency.

You can find more about Good Samaritan laws and whether they exist in your state by contacting a lawyer or your local library.

GOOD SAMARITANS

Check with a lawyer or other legal resource regarding whether AED use is covered by Good Samaritan laws in your state.

A TO Z LISTINGS OF FIRST AID TOPICS

ABDOMINAL PAIN

The abdomen is the area from the nipple line to the groin (the fold where the lower abdomen meets the inner part of the thigh).

Pain in the abdomen can be caused by many different conditions—some minor, others more serious and requiring immediate medical attention. Gastroenteritis (inflammation of the stomach and intestines), appendicitis (inflammation of the appendix), and lactose intolerance (difficulty digesting milk and milk products) are just a few causes of abdominal pain. Sometimes the cause, such as a urinary tract infection, isn't related to the digestive system at all.

By assessing the location of the victim's abdominal pain and identifying other related warning signs, you can quickly tell if the victim requires immediate medical care and help stop abdominal problems from becoming either serious or life-threatening.

What To Look For
•Location of abdominal pain and swollen or rigid abdomen
•Radiation of the pain to the back, neck, jaw, left shoulder, or arm
•Additional symptoms
  •Fever, nausea, and vomiting or diarrhea
  •Internal bleeding—black, tarry stools, vomiting of blood, or bruising on the abdomen
  •Difficulty swallowing
•History of cardiovascular (heart or blood vessel) disease
•Current pregnancy

DID YOU KNOW...

Pain in the abdomen can be caused by many different conditions, some of them not related to the digestive system at all.

A

CHECK

AIRWAY

BREATHING

CIRCULATION

CHECK

AIRWAY

BREATHING

CIRCULATION

What To Do (and Not To Do)

•Check victim's ABCs and treat as necessary (see page 9).

•Call 911 (EMS) immediately if

•Abdominal pain is severe or does not subside.

•Pain is spreading to the victim's back, neck, jaw, left shoulder, or arm—this could be a sign of a heart problem.

•There is severe or sudden pain that feels worse with swallowing (not due to a sore throat), bending, or lying down.

•The abdomen is swollen or rigid.

•The victim either feels faint or is losing consciousness.

•There are any signs of internal bleeding, such as black, tarry stools, vomiting of blood, or bruising on the abdomen.

•There is fever or continuous vomiting or diarrhea.

•The victim is or may be pregnant; abdominal pain may be a sign of a ruptured fallopian tube caused by an ectopic pregnancy (pregnancy that develops outside the uterus).

•You know that the victim has vascular disease.

•If the victim loses consciousness, check his or her ABCs again (see page 9) and treat as necessary.

•Find out as much as you can about the victim's abdominal pain. This information can be given to the doctor or EMS and will help them discover the cause of the pain. If possible, ask the victim

•Where is the pain?

•When did it start?

•What is the pain like? Is it sharp, burning, dull, or crampy? Is the pain constant or does it come and go?

•Is the pain better with belching or passing gas?

•Have the victim lie down in a comfortable position.

• Vomiting can happen at any time, so keep a container, such as a pail or pot, and a damp cloth nearby.

• Applying heat to the abdomen may help relieve the pain. Place a covered hot water bottle on the victim's abdomen.

• *AVOID* giving the victim food or drink until you have consulted a doctor.

• *AVOID* giving medication, an enema, or a laxative to a person with abdominal pain, unless you have been instructed to do so by a doctor.

ALCOHOL ABUSE

Alcohol is the most commonly abused drug in the United States today. Alcohol abuse causes more than 200,000 deaths per year and is the leading cause of serious injuries and accidents.

Alcohol is a depressant, meaning it slows down or hampers a person's responses, coordination, thinking, and judgment. Although alcohol consumption is a socially acceptable practice, alcohol is a drug and an overdose of alcohol may cause blackouts and seizures. Breathing may stop, and the central nervous system may be damaged.

Helping a person who has consumed too much alcohol can be a challenge, as he can be aggressive or nonresponsive. Still, your first aid help may make a big difference to the victim and help him avoid long-term consequences of alcohol dependence.

What To Look For
• Strong smell of alcohol on the breath or clothing
• Staggering or unsteady gait
• Slow reflexes
• Slurred speech
• Deep, noisy breathing that may become shallow
• Rapid, weak pulse
• Sweaty, flushed face
• Nausea and vomiting
• Unusual or unreasonable behavior
• Drowsiness
• Unconsciousness

FOR MORE INFORMATION...

Many organizations, such as Alcoholics Anonymous, offer information and help to combat alcoholism. See page 239.

A

CHECK
_____

AIRWAY

BREATHING

CIRCULATION

What To Do (and Not To Do)

•Check the victim's ABCs and treat as necessary (see page 9).

•Call 911 (EMS).

•Assess the victim for any injuries. This may be difficult, as an intoxicated person may not feel any pain.

•*AVOID* moving the victim if a spinal cord injury is suspected. See Spinal Injury, page 154.

•If the victim is lying down, turn him on his left side—this is called the recovery position and will help prevent further vomiting and allow fluids to drain from his mouth (see page 11).

•Wait with the victim until EMS arrive. Comfort and reassure the victim to help keep him calm. Keep an eye out for changes in behavior, which may change as the alcohol is further absorbed into the bloodstream. *DO NOT* stay with the victim if he becomes violent. You must consider your own safety as well. Move to a safer place and then call the police.

•Try to determine whether the victim has also taken drugs with the alcohol. Look for empty bottles or containers on or near the person. Mixing drugs and alcohol is very dangerous. If you suspect this has occurred, be sure to tell EMS.

•If the victim has been out in the cold for some time, hypothermia (low body temperature, see page 117) may be possible. Move the victim to a warmer place (unless he isn't breathing or may have a spinal injury), remove any wet clothing, and wrap him in warm blankets.

•Be aware that the victim may experience withdrawal from alcohol 12 to 24 hours after the last drink. He may have tremors and be unable to eat or sleep. Be sure to seek medical advice if this occurs. In some victims, delirium tremens (DTs) or rum fits may occur 2 to 5 days after the last drink. Signs of DTs are fever, disorientation, severe tremors, and hallucinations. If you notice any of these signs, call EMS immediately.

ALLERGIC REACTIONS

When our bodies come into contact with a foreign substance, our natural defense system (immune system) works to protect us and destroy the substance. Usually, the immune system does not react to harmless substances (such as pollen or certain foods). But in people with allergies, it mistakenly attacks these substances, causing an allergic reaction.

Many things can cause an allergic reaction, including cosmetics, perfumes, detergents, food, preservatives, medications, insect stings and bites, pollen, dust, and pet dander.

Some allergic reactions are mild; others are more serious (see also Asthma Attack, page 35). Anaphylactic shock, a type of severe allergic reaction, can cause swelling of the airway, interfering with the ability to breathe. It may also lead to a dangerously low blood pressure. If untreated, anaphylactic shock is life-threatening. The good news is that quick action can save a life.

What To Look For

MILD ALLERGIC REACTION
- Itchy, watery eyes
- Runny nose with clear nasal discharge
- Sneezing
- Rash

SEVERE ALLERGIC REACTION
- Flushing in the face, neck, hands, feet, or tongue
- Tongue and lip swelling
- Hives (blotchy, raised rash)
- Tightness in the chest or throat
- Rapid breathing
- Skin around the mouth and lips is blue (see also page 15)
- Nausea and/or vomiting
- Abdominal pain
- Pale, damp skin
- Anxiety

FOR MORE INFORMATION...

Organizations, such as the American Academy of Allergy, Asthma, and Immunology, offer a wealth of information on allergic reactions. See page 240.

A

ANAPHYLACTIC SHOCK

Any of the above signs of severe allergic reaction plus the following:

•Wheezing or difficulty breathing
•Feeling faint, drowsiness
•Loss of consciousness

What To Do (and Not To Do)

MILD ALLERGIC REACTION

•Avoidance of the allergen is the best tactic. Find out what's causing the allergic reaction, and have the victim stay well clear of it.

•Use an allergy medication (either prescription or over-the-counter) as advised by the victim's doctor. This medication can treat mild allergic symptoms like itchy eyes or runny nose.

•Itchy rash may be relieved by cold compresses.

SEVERE ALLERGIC REACTION OR ANAPHYLACTIC SHOCK

•Check the victim's ABCs and treat as necessary (see page 9).

•Call 911 (EMS). Look for a card or identification bracelet that contains information about the victim's allergies.

•If an epinephrine kit is available, inject epinephrine according to instructions. More than one dose may be needed to reverse the anaphylactic shock.

•To help prevent shock, lay the victim down with legs elevated (this will increase blood flow to the heart and brain), and keep him warm with a blanket or coat (see page 145). *DO NOT* use the shock position if the victim is having trouble breathing. Place him in a sitting position instead. *AVOID* moving the victim if a spinal cord injury is suspected (see page 154).

•If the victim has been stung by a bee, search for the bee's stinger in the skin and remove it. Scrape the stinger away with your fingernail, a knife blade, or a credit card. *DO NOT* use tweezers. A stinger will release more poison if it is squeezed by tweez-

CHECK

AIRWAY
BREATHING
CIRCULATION

ers. Using soap and water, wash the sting site and cover it with a cold compress or ice pack. If possible, position the victim so that the sting site is below the level of his heart.

•Comfort the victim and help him stay calm while you're waiting for EMS.

•*AVOID* giving the victim food or drink until you have consulted a doctor.

ALTITUDE SICKNESS (MOUNTAIN SICKNESS)

Altitude sickness is caused by insufficient oxygen at high altitudes, usually above 8,000 feet. It can be mild and treated by simple measures, or it can be more severe, requiring immediate, lifesaving action.

There are two types of severe altitude sickness. In high-altitude pulmonary edema (HAPE), fluid collects in the lungs and interferes with breathing. In high-altitude cerebral edema (HACE), fluid builds up in the brain, causing swelling and hindering brain function. With prompt descent to a lower altitude and treatment, most people with severe altitude sickness will recover. But ignoring or failing to treat this condition can lead to severe problems.

What To Look For

MILD ALTITUDE SICKNESS
•Headache
•Shortness of breath
•Tiredness
•Swelling of the face, arms, and legs
•Nausea and vomiting
•Difficulty sleeping

SEVERE ALTITUDE SICKNESS

HAPE (HIGH-ALTITUDE PULMONARY EDEMA)
•Shortness of breath

PREVENTION POINTERS

There are steps you can take to prevent altitude sickness altogether, such as climbing slowly and stopping to rest whenever you feel tired or out of breath. Some prescription medications—acetazolamide (Diamox) and dexamethasone (Decadron)—can help too. (For more on How to Prevent Altitude Sickness, see page 211.)

A

•Breathing that gurgles or rattles
•Cough with pink, frothy discharge (signs of bleeding)
•Rapid pulse (more than 100 beats per minute)
•Skin around the mouth and lips is blue (see also page 15)
•Headache
•Chest tightness

HACE (HIGH-ALTITUDE CEREBRAL EDEMA)
•Severe headache
•Difficulty walking
•Nausea and vomiting
•Extreme tiredness
•Hallucinations
•Confusion and irritability
•Loss of consciousness
•Coma

What To Do (and Not To Do)

MILD ALTITUDE SICKNESS
•Tell the victim to rest. He should *NOT* climb any further.
•Give the victim fluids and aspirin or acetaminophen.
•Make sure the victim does not smoke or drink alcohol—both can make symptoms more severe.
•Monitor the victim's condition. If symptoms do not improve, he should descend and seek immediate medical care. If the symptoms are completely gone, the victim may begin ascending again.

SEVERE ALTITUDE SICKNESS
•Check the victim's ABCs and treat as necessary (see page 9).
•Seek emergency medical attention.
•Immediately help the victim to descend at least 1,000 feet.
•Place the victim in a sitting position to ease breathing. Calm the victim, and keep him warm.

CHECK

AIRWAY
BREATHING
CIRCULATION

AMPUTATION

See Severed Limb, page 141

ANKLE SPRAIN

See Strains and Sprains, page 157

ASTHMA ATTACK

Asthma is a condition—often lifelong—that affects the ability of airways to carry air to and from the lungs. When a person with asthma is exposed to certain irritants (such as cigarette smoke, cold air, or pollution), his airways become swollen and inflamed, blocking the flow of air and making breathing difficult.

Many asthma attacks develop slowly, so medication can be taken to reverse them. If an attack develops more quickly and is not treated properly, it can become serious and potentially life-threatening. Fortunately, most severe asthma attacks can be treated with prompt and proper action.

What's more, people can learn to predict and prevent these attacks from occurring again. Using a peak flow meter, for instance, is an important preventive tool that measures the maximum rate at which air is exhaled from the lungs. This meter helps keep track of changes in breathing and can signal a possible asthma attack in its early stages.

> ## FOR MORE INFORMATION...
>
> Organizations—such as the American Academy of Allergy, Asthma, and Immunology—offer a wide range of information on asthma. See page 240.

What To Look For

MILD TO MODERATE ATTACK
- Breathing that is difficult and faster than usual
- Reduced ability to exhale
- Wheezing
- Tightness in the chest
- Flaring nostrils

•Dry cough, especially at night
•Increased pulse
•Pale, clammy skin
•Anxiety
•Vomiting
•Fever
•Drowsiness, poor concentration
•Reduced peak flow rate (maximum rate that air is exhaled from lungs, as measured on the victim's peak flow meter)

SEVERE ATTACK
•Asthma medication produces no response or is needed more than every 4 hours
•Bluish tinge to the skin (sign of lack of oxygen in the blood) (see also page 15)
•Rapid pulse (over 120 beats per minute)
•Breathing becomes more difficult or inaudible (this means the victim is not moving enough air to make any noise)
•Inability to cough
•Peak flow rate is less than 50% of victim's personal best (as measured on the victim's peak flow meter)
•Collapse and unconsciousness

What To Do (and Not To Do)

MILD TO MODERATE ATTACK
•Check the victim's ABCs and treat as necessary (see page 9).
•Calm the victim and place him in a comfortable, sitting position. Loosen any tight clothing, and remove rings and any other constricting jewelry.
•People with asthma often have action plans (provided by their doctor) for dealing with asthma attacks. Ask the victim if he has an action plan. If so, follow the instructions.
•Ask the victim about his asthma medication. If available, give four puffs of the victim's bronchodilator, then one puff per minute (up to a total of eight puffs) to relieve symptoms. This medica-

CHECK

AIRWAY
BREATHING
CIRCULATION

tion will help widen the airways, so breathing is easier. If the medication does not relieve the attack, call EMS (if this has not already been done). *AVOID* giving any medication that has not been prescribed by the victim's doctor.

•If this is the victim's first asthma attack and medication is not available, call EMS (if this has not already been done).

•While waiting for EMS, continue to calm the victim. Stress or anxiety can increase the severity of an asthma attack.

•When EMS arrive, have the victim take his medication with him to show the doctor what he is taking for his attacks.

•Try to determine what triggered the attack. This information is important to help prevent future asthma attacks.

SEVERE ATTACK

•Do not delay getting help. Call 911 (EMS) immediately.

•Inject the victim with epinephrine, if available, according to his doctor's instructions.

•Ask the victim if he has an action plan for dealing with severe asthma attacks. If so, follow the instructions.

•Ask the victim about his asthma medication. If available, give four puffs of the victim's bronchodilator, then one puff per minute (up to a total of eight puffs) to relieve symptoms. This medication will help widen airways, so breathing is easier. *AVOID* giving any medication that has not been prescribed by the victim's doctor.

•While waiting for EMS, comfort the victim. Stress or anxiety can increase the severity of an asthma attack.

•When EMS arrive, have the victim take his medication with him to show the doctor what he is taking for his attacks.

•Try to determine what triggered the attack. This information is important to help prevent future severe asthma attacks.

BEE STINGS

See Insect Stings, page 118

BITES

Bite injuries are caused by a wide range of animals—from cats and dogs to snakes and spiders. Other animals, such as bees and marine life, can sting. Some bites or stings can be minor, needing only proper cleaning to control infection. Others can pose greater risks, such as tetanus, rabies, tissue damage, or severe allergic reaction—all requiring immediate medical care.

Treatment will depend on the animal that has bitten the victim. So be sure to refer to the specific type of bite the victim has experienced.

See Cat, Dog, and Other Animal Bites (page 56), Insect Stings (page 118), Marine Animal Bites and Stings (page 121), Rabies (page 136), Scorpion Stings (page 137), Snake Bites (page 149), Spider Bites (page 152), and Tick Bites (page 166).

PREVENTION POINTERS

Whenever blood is present at the scene of an emergency, there is a risk of transmitting certain viral diseases from rescuer to victim or vice versa. That's why it's vital to take steps such as washing your hands and wearing gloves, if available. By following these and other precautions, you will be protecting yourself and the victim from possible illness (see Precautions and Guidelines for the Rescuer, page 24).

BLEEDING—EXTERNAL

External bleeding occurs when the skin is cut and a blood vessel is damaged. The severity of the resulting injury is determined by the cut's depth, the type of blood vessel damaged, and the time taken to control the bleeding. Be aware that the amount of bleeding is not a good way to judge an injury's severity—serious injuries don't always bleed heavily.

There are three different types of bleeding—arterial (bright red blood that spurts with each heartbeat from damaged arteries), venous (dark red blood that comes from veins), and capillary bleeding (blood that oozes from tiny blood vessels found throughout the body).

No matter what type of bleeding you are faced with, the methods to control it are the same.

See also Bleeding—Internal, page 41.

What To Look For

- Bleeding from an open wound
- Rapid, weak pulse
- Pale, cold, clammy skin
- Sweating
- Skin around the mouth and lips is blue (see also page 15)
- Shock (see page 146)

What To Do (and Not To Do)

- Wash your hands with soap and water. Wear gloves if available.
- Locate the site of the bleeding. If necessary, remove or cut the victim's clothing.

IF THE BLEEDING IS NOT SEVERE

- Wash the wound with soap and water.
- Apply direct pressure to stop the bleeding, and cover with a clean, dry dressing.

IF THE BLEEDING IS SEVERE

- Check the victim's ABCs and treat as necessary (see page 9).
- Call 911 (EMS).
- To help prevent shock, lay the victim down with legs elevated (this will increase blood flow to the heart and brain) and keep him warm with a blanket or coat (see page 147). *AVOID* moving the victim if a spinal cord injury is suspected (see page 154).
- *DO NOT* remove an object that is embedded in a wound.
- *DO NOT* wash wounds that are deep and bleeding, since this might increase or restart bleeding.
- Place a sterile pad or clean cloth over the wound and apply direct, constant pressure. *DO NOT* apply direct pressure if an embedded object or a protruding bone is present; press down firmly on either side of the injury.
- If bleeding doesn't stop, apply harder pressure with both hands over a greater area. *DO NOT* remove blood-stained dressings; instead, place another dressing on top to soak up the blood.

CHECK

AIRWAY

BREATHING

CIRCULATION

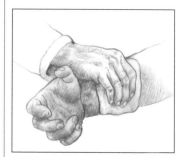

Applying direct pressure to a wound.

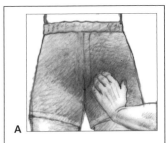

A

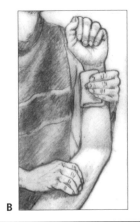

B

Location of major pressure points. (A) If bleeding from a leg wound cannot be stopped by direct compression and elevation, the femoral artery in the groin can be compressed to limit blood flow to the leg. (B) Likewise, the brachial artery in the upper arm, between the armpit and elbow, can be compressed to limit blood flow to the rest of the arm.

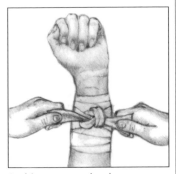

Applying a pressure bandage.

• If possible, elevate the wound above the victim's heart level, while still maintaining the pressure.

• If the bleeding continues, call EMS (if this has not already been done). Then apply pressure at the victim's pressure points (where a blood vessel is near the skin's surface and close to a bone). This will limit blood flow to the injury. There are two major pressure points:

  • The *femoral artery* in the groin, where the lower abdomen meets the inner part of the thigh (use for a leg injury): Feel for a pulse in the groin. Then, using your fingers and with your arm extended straight, press the artery against the pelvic bone until you can't feel a pulse. Use both hands if necessary.

  • The *brachial artery* on the upper inside arm (use for arm injuries): You can find it by feeling for a pulse below the round muscle of the biceps, halfway between the armpit and elbow. Using your fingers, press the artery until you can't feel a pulse.

• After the bleeding stops, or to free your hands to check for other injuries, apply a pressure bandage. While pulling steadily, wrap a roller gauze bandage or long cloth tightly over the dressing, and above and below the wound. Split the bandage end into two strips, then knot the ends tightly, directly over the wound. A pressure bandage should be tight enough to keep pressure on the wound but not so tight that it cuts off circulation. A bandage is too tight if there is no pulse beyond the wound (away from the victim's trunk) or if the skin in that area is turning blue.

• In general, a tourniquet (a strip of material placed tightly around a limb to stop the flow of blood) is *NOT* recommended, as it might damage nerves and blood vessels.

• Calm the victim and stay with him until EMS has arrived.

BLEEDING—INTERNAL

To most of us, bleeding involves the sight of red blood oozing from an open wound. But bleeding can also occur inside our bodies, without visible blood or broken skin. For this reason, internal bleeding can be hard to detect.

Internal bleeding is not a disease but a sign of an internal injury or illness. It may be a sign of a serious problem (such as a traumatic injury) or a minor one (such as a bladder infection).

Internal bleeding may show itself in different ways, including blood in the stool, vomit, urine, vagina, and severe bruising on the body. Whatever the source, it is important to seek medical attention to identify and treat it.

See also Bloody Stool (page 43), Bloody Urine (page 45), Bloody Vomit (page 46), and Vaginal Bleeding (page 169).

What To Look For
- Dark red blood mixed with the stool
- Bright red blood covering the stool
- Black or tarry stool
- Bright red blood in the urine
- Urine that looks like "cola"
- Urine that is smoky in appearance
- Vomit that looks like coffee grounds
- Evidence that an injury has occurred
- Abdominal pain
- Swollen or rigid abdomen
- Nausea and vomiting
- Shortness of breath
- Faintness
- Pale, cool, clammy skin

What To Do (and Not To Do)
- Check the victim's ABCs and treat as necessary (see page 9).

CHECK

Airway

Breathing

Circulation

•Call 911 (EMS) immediately if

> •Sudden, massive bleeding occurs in the stool, urine, vomit, or vagina
>
> •Abdominal pain is severe or does not subside
>
> •The abdomen is swollen or rigid
>
> •There is fever, continuous vomiting, or diarrhea
>
> •There are signs of severe injury, including open wounds or severe bruising
>
> •The victim either feels faint or is losing consciousness

•To help prevent shock, lay the victim down with legs elevated (this will increase blood flow to the heart and brain) and keep him warm with a blanket or coat (see page 147). *AVOID* moving the victim if a spinal cord injury is suspected (see page 154).

•Vomiting can happen at any time, so keep a container, such as a pail or pot, and a damp cloth nearby.

•Have the victim lie on his left side—this is called the recovery position (see page 11). It will help prevent further vomiting and allow fluids to drain from his mouth.

•*DO NOT* give a medication to a person who may be suffering from internal bleeding, except if advised by a doctor.

•*DO NOT* give the victim food or drink.

•If this is not an emergency situation, be sure to follow up with the victim's doctor. The source of the bleeding must be identified and treated.

BLISTERS

Blisters form when an area of the outer skin separates from the under layer, forming a pocket where clear fluid gathers. If a small blood vessel breaks as the blister forms, the pocket will contain blood instead.

Blisters can be caused by friction (for example, from ill-fitting shoes) or by chemical or heat burns. In almost all cases, a blister should be left to heal on its own, although a friction blister may be drained if it is large and interferes with the use of hands or feet. When treated properly, blisters will heal quickly.

What To Look For
• Pocket of clear fluid or blood under the top layer of skin
• Sensitivity or mild pain in the blister area when pressure is applied
• Redness and swelling

What To Do (and Not To Do)
• Most blisters, particularly those caused by burns, should be left alone. The outer layer of the blister provides sterile protection. If not popped or cut, the blister will usually heal by itself. The body will slowly absorb the fluid or blood, and the blister will fall off.
• In the meantime, keep the blister area clean. Cover it with a bandage if the blister is being rubbed or irritated.
• If the blister pops on its own, wash the area with an antibacterial soap and cover with a bandage.

DRAINING A LARGE FRICTION BLISTER
• Clean the area with antibacterial soap. Pat dry and wipe thoroughly with rubbing alcohol.
• Using a sterile needle, poke holes in the blister at several places. Gently press the blister to squeeze out the fluid. *DO NOT* remove the skin. Allow it to provide a protective cover.
• Apply antibiotic cream and cover with a bandage.
• Repeat these steps if the blister returns.
• If the blister is very large and painful, or signs of infection develop (swelling, fever, or red streaks), seek medical care.

BLOODY STOOL

We may not relish the task of stool inspection, but it's wise to do it on a regular basis. That way any problems, such as bleeding, can be discovered early.

PREVENTION POINTERS

You can prevent blisters by wearing shoes and socks that fit properly; by wearing the appropriate gloves for activities, such as gardening, that involve working with tools; and by covering areas exposed to rubbing (caused by sandal straps, for instance) with moleskin or adhesive bandages.

B

B

Blood in the stool is a sign of an internal problem brought on by illness or injury. Most causes of bleeding are not serious—such as hemorrhoids—and can be easily treated.

You can help the victim by encouraging him to seek a doctor's advice. It's important to identify the source of blood in the stool.

What To Look For

- Dark red blood mixed with the stool
- Bright red blood covering the stool
- Black or tarry stool
- Evidence that an injury has occurred
- Bruising on the abdomen
- Use of blood thinners
- Abdominal pain
- Swollen or rigid abdomen
- Nausea and vomiting
- Shortness of breath
- Dizziness and faintness
- Pale, cool, clammy skin
- Loss of consciousness

What To Do (and Not To Do)

- Check the victim's ABCs and treat as necessary (see page 9).
- Call 911 (EMS) immediately if
  - Sudden, massive bleeding occurs in the stool.
  - Abdominal pain is severe or does not subside.
  - The abdomen is swollen or rigid.
  - There is fever, constant vomiting, or diarrhea.
  - The victim either feels faint or is losing consciousness.
- To help prevent shock, lay the victim down with legs elevated (this will increase blood flow to the heart and brain) and keep him warm with a blanket or coat (see page 147). *AVOID* moving the victim if a spinal cord injury is suspected (see page 154).

CHECK

Airway

Breathing

Circulation

•Vomiting can happen at any time, so keep a container, such as a pail or pot, and a damp cloth nearby.

•Have the victim lie on his left side—this is called the recovery position (see page 11). It will help prevent further vomiting and allow fluids to drain from his mouth.

•*AVOID* giving medication, an enema, or a laxative to a person with bloody stool, unless instructed by a medical doctor.

•Calm the victim and stay with him until EMS arrives.

•If this is not an emergency situation, be sure to follow up with the victim's doctor. The source of the bleeding must be identified and treated.

BLOODY URINE

Blood in the urine (hematuria) is not always easy to detect. While red blood may be visible, sometimes the urine may be the color of cola or, if there is less blood, it may have a smoky appearance.

Bloody urine has many causes—some are minor (such as strenuous exercise); other causes are more serious (such as kidney disease, abdominal injury, or bladder tumors).

Whenever blood is noticed in the urine, seek medical care. It's important to identify the source, no matter how minor it might be. Your prompt action will help protect the victim's well-being.

What To Look For
•Bright red blood present in the urine
•Urine looks like cola
•Urine is smoky in appearance
•Bruising or open wounds on the abdomen
•Use of blood thinners
•Abdominal pain
•Swollen or rigid abdomen
•Back or bladder pain
•Nausea

DID YOU KNOW...
Blood in the urine may sometimes be the color of cola or have a smoky appearance.

•Swelling of the face, or ankles, or both
•Fever
•Shortness of breath
•Dizziness and faintness
•Pale, cool, clammy skin
•Loss of consciousness

What To Do (and Not To Do)

•If there is severe, massive bleeding in the urine

   •Check the victim's ABCs and treat as necessary (see page 9).

   •Call 911 (EMS) or go to the emergency room.

   •To help prevent shock, lay the victim down with legs elevated (this will increase blood flow to the heart and brain) and keep him warm with a blanket or coat (see page 147). *AVOID* moving the victim if a spinal cord injury is suspected (see page 154).

•Vomiting can happen at any time, so keep a container, such as a pail or pot, and a damp cloth nearby.

•Have the victim lie on his left side—this is called the recovery position (see page 11). It will help prevent further vomiting and allow fluids to drain from his mouth.

•*AVOID* giving any medication to the victim, unless instructed by a doctor.

•Calm the victim and stay with him until EMS arrive.

•If the bleeding is not severe, be sure to follow up with the victim's doctor. The source must be identified and treated.

CHECK

AIRWAY
BREATHING
CIRCULATION

BLOODY VOMIT

Bloody vomit can indicate a serious condition, such as abdominal injury, liver disease, blood-clotting problems, and drug or alcohol overdose.

   Whenever a victim vomits blood, seek immediate medical attention. Acting quickly will safeguard his health and help prevent long-term problems.

What To Look For
•Vomit that looks like coffee grounds
•Bruising on the chest or abdomen
•Use of blood thinners
•Chest or abdominal pain
•Swollen or rigid abdomen
•Nausea
•Fever
•Shortness of breath
•Dizziness and faintness
•Pale, cool, clammy skin
•Loss of consciousness

What To Do (and Not To Do)
•Check the victim's ABCs and treat as necessary (see page 9).
•Call 911 (EMS).
•To help prevent shock, lay the victim down with his legs elevated (this will increase blood flow to the heart and brain) and keep him warm with a blanket or coat (see page 147). *AVOID* moving the victim if a spinal cord injury is suspected (for more details, see page 154).
•Keep a container, such as a pail or pot, and a damp cloth nearby.
•Have the victim lie on his left side—this is called the recovery position (see page 11). It will help prevent further vomiting and allow fluids to drain from his mouth.
•*DO NOT* give a medication to a person with bloody vomit, unless instructed by a doctor.
•*DO NOT* give the victim food or drink.
•Calm the victim and stay with him until the arrival of EMS.

> **CHECK**
>
> Airway
> Breathing
> Circulation

BREATHING EMERGENCIES

Oxygen is essential to life—each and every one of the cells in your body needs oxygen to function.

You bring oxygen into your body by breathing air into your lungs. From there, the oxygen enters your bloodstream and circulates throughout your body. It's equally important to expel the used air—which carries waste products from the blood in the form of carbon dioxide—by breathing out.

It is the respiratory system, made up of your nose, mouth, windpipe, lungs, and blood vessels, that carries out this important process. To breathe properly, your respiratory system must be in good working order. However, it is vulnerable to sudden illness, injury, and chronic (long-term) conditions.

Whenever breathing emergencies arise, recognize them and seek immediate medical care. By doing so, you can help save lives.
See also Allergic Reactions (page 31), Asthma Attack (page 35), Burns (page 54), Choking (page 67), Drowning (page 84), Head Injury (page 107), Heart Attack (page 111), Hyperventilation (page 116), and Smoke Inhalation (page 148).

What To Look For
•Breathing rate either above or below normal levels—normally, adults breathe at 10 to 20 breaths per minute, children 20 to 25 breaths per minute, and infants 30 to 40 breaths per minute.
•Shallow, irregular breathing
•Chest pain
•Tightness in the chest
•Stridor (difficulty getting air into the lungs)
•Wheezing (difficulty getting air out of the lungs)
•Difficulty speaking due to lack of breath
•Flaring of the nostrils
•Pursed lips
•Hoarse, barking cough (this is the main symptom of croup—see page 49)
•Anxiety, dizziness, or confusion
•Numbness or tingling in the hands and feet
•Fainting

B

What To Do (and Not To Do)

•Check the victim's ABCs and treat as necessary (see page 9).

•Call 911 (EMS).

•Calm the victim and place him or her in a comfortable, sitting position, if possible. *AVOID* moving the victim if a spinal cord injury is suspected (see Spinal Injury, page 154).

•If the victim has asthma, treat as necessary (see page 35).

•If the victim is choking, attempt to remove the obstruction with abdominal or chest thrusts (see page 67).

CHEST INJURY

IF THE VICTIM HAS A CHEST INJURY

•Check the victim's ABCs and treat as necessary (see page 9).

•Call 911 (EMS).

•*For a sucking wound* (air entering the chest through a penetrating wound): Tape a plastic bag or wrap (or anything else available) to the wound to prevent air from entering the chest. Leave one side untaped for air to get out.

•*For a rib fracture:* Support the ribs and chest by placing a soft object (such as a pillow) against the injured area and secure with bandages.

•*For an embedded object:* Hold the object in place with bulky padding and secure with bandages. *DO NOT* remove any object that is embedded in a chest wound.

CROUP

Croup refers to breathing difficulties in children caused by swelling in the upper airway passages. It is characterized by a barking cough. If a child has croup but is breathing normally between bouts of coughing

•Take the child into the bathroom. Close the door and fill the room with steam by running a hot shower. Sit in the room, but *NOT* in the shower, for 15 to 20 minutes.

CHECK

AIRWAY

BREATHING

CIRCULATION

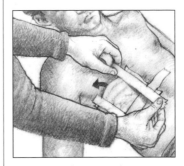

Covering a sucking wound.

B

• If steam doesn't work, take the child outside into moist, cool air.
• *DO NOT* try to open the child's airway with your finger.
• If breathing gets more difficult, call 911 (EMS).
• Stay with the child and reassure him until EMS arrive.

BROKEN BONES

There are more than 200 separate bones in the human skeleton. Any one of these bones can be broken, either directly (where the bone breaks at point of contact) or indirectly (where it breaks at a point away from the point of contact). Broken bones can run the gamut, from a slight crack to serious compound fractures, with a bone broken in several places or protruding through the skin.

By providing the right first aid, such as immobilizing the broken bone, you can do much to reduce the victim's discomfort and help prevent further injury until EMS arrive.

DID YOU KNOW...

Bones break more easily in the elderly, even with a minor fall.

What To Look For
• Recent fall or blow
• Injured limb looks shortened or rotated or is lying at an angle (where there is no joint)
• Tenderness and pain at the injury site that is worse with moving
• Swelling and bruising
• Exposed bones
• Locked joint
• Pale, cool, clammy skin
• Visible wound and bleeding
• Nausea
• Shock (see page 146)

CHECK

Airway

Breathing

Circulation

What To Do (and Not To Do)
• Check the victim's ABCs and treat as necessary (see page 9).

- Call 911 (EMS).
- Remove or cut away victim's clothing covering the wound; remove any of the victim's rings or constricting jewelry.
- If there is bleeding, take steps to control it (see page 38).
- Immobilize the injury by padding it with pillows and towels. If EMS are not nearby and you must transport the victim to the hospital, you may need to splint the broken bone (see Splints, page 52).
- Place the limb, if possible, slightly above the level of the victim's heart.
- *DO NOT* try to straighten a broken bone, unless there is no pulse below the break (this may mean the bone is squeezing an artery and stopping the flow of blood.) For an arm injury, check for a pulse by placing your fingers (*not* your thumb) on the thumb side of the victim's wrist. For a leg injury, place your fingers between the victim's inside ankle bone and Achilles tendon (the tendon at the back of the lower leg that connects to the heel bone).
- If you can't find a pulse, and the limb is colder than the noninjured limb, gently apply traction (tug and straighten the bone) and check if the pulse returns. If it has returned, continue gently applying traction until EMS arrive. If the pulse does not return, apply stronger traction and recheck to see if the pulse returns.

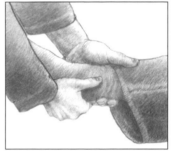

Applying gentle traction to the ankle to straighten a broken bone in the upper leg that is blocking blood flow.

- To reduce swelling around the injury, apply a cold compress or ice pack, but do not allow it to touch the skin directly.
- To help prevent shock, lay the victim down with legs elevated (this will increase blood flow to the heart and brain) and keep him warm with a blanket or coat (see page 147). *AVOID* moving the victim if a spinal cord injury is suspected (for more details, see page 154).
- Keep the victim still. If the victim must be moved (because of a dangerous situation, for instance), drag him by the clothes, keeping the head in line with the body. Drag the victim forward or backward, never sideways.

SPLINTS

A splint is a flexible or rigid device that protects and immobilizes an injury like a broken bone. Some of the common splints are described below. To better understand how to apply all types of splints, take a course from a first aid organization, such as the American Red Cross or the National Safety Council.

GENERAL RULES
•Apply a splint to the injury in the same position you found it in.
•While you're applying the splint, support the injured limb with your hands (or better yet, have someone help you).
•If you suspect a broken bone, apply the splint both above and below the break.
•If a joint appears to have been broken, splint the bones above and below it.
•To make a rigid splint, you may use a variety of materials found in your home, such as umbrellas, boards, rake handles, or rolled newspapers. If you can't find a suitable splint, you can secure the injured limb to another uninjured part of the body or to the victim's clothing. You might, for instance, roll the bottom edge of a shirt around an injured arm and pin it up to the shirt.
•Rigid splints may cause some discomfort

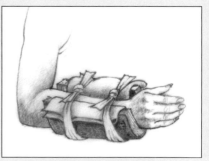

Splint for a broken arm. A folded magazine with padding can be used to make the splint, which is tied in place above and below the suspected break.

for the victim. If possible, apply soft padding between the limb and the splint.

INJURED ARM
Use a sling to support the splinted arm (see illustration below):
•Get or cut a large triangle of cloth.
•Place the injured arm at right angles with the palm facing in and the thumb facing upward. Support this arm while you apply the splint.
•The long side of the triangle should run vertically, closest to the hand. You should place

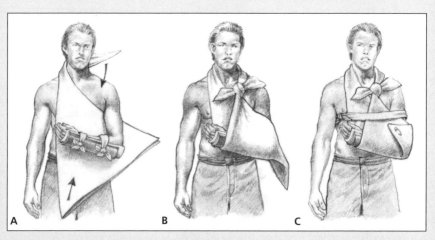

Applying a sling to support a splinted arm. (A) Positioning the arm on the sling. (B) Tying the sling. (C) Binding the sling to the body.

SPLINTS *(continued)*

it over the hand of the injured arm, with the fingers showing.
•Place the opposite point under the elbow of the injured arm.
•Pull the top corner over the victim's shoulder on the uninjured side. Pull up the bottom corner over the other shoulder. Knot the two corners together.
•Pin up any extra cloth at the elbow.
•You may bind the sling to the body by wrapping a piece of cloth around the victim's chest and knotting it at the uninjured side.

INJURED ANKLE
An injured ankle can be immobilized in a soft, flexible splint:
•Place a pillow or soft blanket under the ankle, so that it extends from midcalf to beyond the foot.
•Wrap the pillow or blanket around the ankle and tie it twice.

•Place a pillow or other support under the ankle to keep it elevated.

INJURED LOWER LEG OR KNEE
Either a rigid or soft splint can be used, depending on what materials you have on hand.
•Find two long boards (or other rigid material). One board is for the outside of the injured leg and must be long enough to extend from the victim's waist to beyond the foot. The other board will lie on the inside of the injured leg and should be long enough to extend from the groin (where the lower abdomen meets the inner part of the thigh) to beyond the foot.
•Place the boards on the inner and outer part of the injured leg. Place some soft padding between the boards and the leg and tie the splint in three or four places.

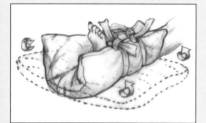

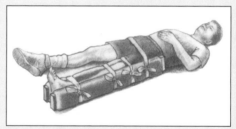

•Fold up the pillow or blanket around the foot, with toes showing, and tie it once near the end.

•If you don't have rigid materials, roll up a blanket and place it between the victim's legs. Tie the legs together in three or four places.

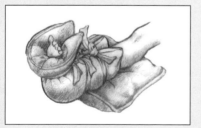

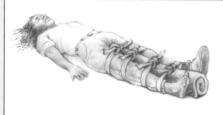

•While you're waiting for EMS, calm the victim and try to make him as comfortable as possible. *DO NOT* give food or drink to the victim.

BURNS

Burn injuries come from a variety of sources—heat (both wet and dry), chemicals, smoke, electrical current, lightning, and the sun.

The severity of a burn depends on its size, location, and depth.

SIZE
The larger the burn area on a victim, the more serious the burn.

LOCATION
Burns to the feet, hands, face, airway, and genitals are usually considered more serious.

DEPTH
The deeper the burn, the more serious it is. Previously, burn depth was classified as first, second, and third degree. Now, it's more commonly described as superficial (minor damage to the top layer of skin), partial thickness (skin is damaged but its full depth is not completely destroyed), and full thickness (full depth of skin, hair follicles, muscles, nerves, bones, or internal organs are damaged or destroyed).

How you respond to a burn injury will be determined by the type of burn and its severity. But here's a good rule of thumb for all burns—immediate action by stopping the burning and cooling the burn with water will help limit the damage to the victim.

See Chemical Burns (page 58), Electrical Burns (page 90), Sunburn (page 161), and Thermal Burns (page 164).

CARBON MONOXIDE AND OTHER TOXIC FUMES

Gases and fumes are all around us; they are not a concern unless you are exposed to them in poorly ventilated rooms, garages, and other spaces.

Carbon monoxide (CO) is produced by appliances or heaters that burn gas, oil, wood, propane, or kerosene. Dangerous levels can occur when these fuels aren't completely burned and vented, as can happen with faulty space heaters, furnaces, and water heaters and plugged chimneys or vents. You can even be at risk outside the home—leaving the car running in a closed garage or riding in the back of an enclosed pick-up truck can expose you to high levels of CO.

You can do a lot to protect your family from exposure to toxic levels of CO. Installing CO alarms (also called detectors or monitors) and maintaining appliances and heaters in your home are some of the simple but effective measures (see page 173).

CO is an invisible, nonirritating toxic gas that has no taste or odor, so it's difficult to know whether people are being exposed to it. Other fumes, like those given off by ammonia and other chemicals, paints, and solvents, have a strong odor and are more readily noticed.

Always be on the lookout for the signs of exposure to carbon monoxide and other toxic fumes. By acting quickly, you can help save a victim from inhalation poisoning.

What To Look For
- Headache
- Dizziness
- Nausea and vomiting
- Blurred vision
- Difficulty breathing
- Weakness
- Chest pain

RADON

Radon, another toxic gas, is produced by the natural breakdown of uranium in rock, soil, and water. This gas moves up from the ground and into the air, where it can seep through cracks and holes in the foundations, floors, and walls and become trapped in your home. Radon doesn't cause immediate health problems, but long-term exposure has been associated with cancer (see page 174).

DID YOU KNOW...

Mixing chlorine and ammonia can produce life-threatening toxic fumes. Always check the labels of your cleaning agents carefully.

B

•Confusion and memory loss

•Loss of consciousness

•Any of the above symptoms that come and go and that worsen when the victim is in a particular area

•People and pets around the victim may appear ill as well

What To Do (and Not To Do)

•Assess how safe it is to enter the area.

•Immediately remove the victim from the exposed area and take him into fresh air. Make sure all other people and pets leave as well.

•Check the victim's ABCs and treat as necessary (see page 9).

•Call 911 (EMS).

•Calm the victim and wait with him until EMS arrive.

CARDIOPULMONARY RESUSCITATION (CPR)

See page 12

CAT, DOG, AND OTHER ANIMAL BITES

Dogs and cats are a common feature of many households; hamsters, rabbits, gerbils, ferrets, and mice are also kept as pets. Domestic animals may be a source of love, companionship, and comfort, but they can also be a source of injury. Wild animals (for example, raccoons) pose a higher risk to victims, as they are more likely to carry the rabies virus.

Dogs and cats are responsible for most injuries caused by animal bites. Dog bites present two main concerns—damage to tissues and infection. Cats bites can cause deep puncture wounds that have a much greater chance of becoming infected.

CHECK

Airway

Breathing

Circulation

Most domestic animal bites are minor and can be easily treated. Others are more serious and may require emergency medical treatment. All bites from wild animals should be treated by a health care professional, since a careful assessment must be made regarding the risk of rabies.

What To Look For

•Bite marks that may have broken the skin
•Redness, swelling, and pain at the bite site, especially 24 to 48 hours after the bite
•Bleeding
•Anxiety and fear

What To Do (and Not To Do)

IF THE WOUND IS SEVERE OR THE VICTIM IS UNCONSCIOUS

•Check the victim's ABCs and treat as necessary (see page 9).
•Call 911 (EMS).
•To help prevent shock, lay the victim down with legs elevated (this will increase blood flow to the heart and brain) and keep him warm with a blanket or coat (see page 147).
•Wash your hands with soap and water.
•Calm the victim, and inspect the wound.
•Clean the wound with soap and water from a hose or faucet at full pressure. Continue rinsing for at least 10 minutes.
•If the skin has not been broken, apply an ice pack or cold compress to ease the pain and swelling.
•If the skin has been broken, stop the bleeding by applying direct pressure (see page 39). Cover the wound with a clean, dry dressing. Seek medical attention so the wound can be cleaned more thoroughly. Depending on the wound, stitches may be needed.
•If possible, elevate the wounded limb above the level of the heart to reduce swelling.
•Try to identify the animal that has bitten the victim. *DO NOT* get near or try to capture it. If you

---

CHECK

Airway
Breathing
Circulation

know the owners, contact them to find out if the animal has been immunized against rabies. Report the biting incident to an animal control group or to the police. If the animal's immunization status is unknown, the animal needs to be watched for rabies (see also Rabies, page 136).

•The victim may need a tetanus shot, antibiotic medication, or rabies vaccination series.

•Afterward, check the victim's wound on a daily basis for signs of infection, such as redness, swelling, or discharge. Also check the victim for fever. If you notice any of these signs, seek medical attention.

CHEMICAL BURNS

A chemical burn is caused by contact with a corrosive chemical (dry or wet). Many chemicals can cause burns—from those found in the home (such as bleach or oven cleaner) to industrial-strength chemicals used in factories.

The signs of chemical burns may take a while to appear, but don't let that fool you. Chemical burns always need immediate attention. Some chemicals continue to burn as long as they are in contact with the skin or eyes. Your prompt action can make all the difference in reducing the burn's damage.

What To Look For
•Victim has come into contact with a chemical
•Severe, stinging pain
•Redness, blisters, and swelling around the burn site (these signs may not be evident right away)

What To Do (and Not To Do)
•Contact your local poison control center.

•Put on protective gloves and, if possible, wear protective eyewear. You need to make sure the chemical doesn't land on you.

•Brush away any dry chemicals. Immediately flood the affected area with cold water for 20 minutes or longer, until the victim no longer feels a burning sensation. *DO NOT* use a hard spray. If the chemi-

PREVENTION POINTERS

Proper handling and storage of chemicals in the home can prevent burns (see page 189 for more information).

WHEN EYES ARE AFFECTED

The eyes are an easy target when chemicals spill, so be sure to provide immediate first aid to prevent long-term damage.

•Hold the eyelid open and use a gentle stream of water to flush it for 20 minutes—this is especially important for burns from alkali substances such as lye.

•Be sure to avoid washing the chemical into the victim's other eye or onto another part of the body.

•*DO NOT* use an eyecup or eyedrops, unless a doctor or EMS tell you to do so.

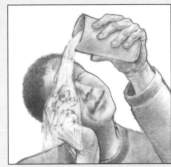

Flushing the eye for a chemical burn.

cal has come into contact with the victim's eyes, see When Eyes Are Affected, above.

•While you're flushing the affected area, remove any of the victim's clothing that may have been exposed to the chemical.

•Wash the burn area with soap and water. Gently dry and cover with a sterile, dry dressing. For large areas, use a clean towel or pillow case. *DO NOT* use neutralizers (such as baking soda or vinegar) in an attempt to counteract the chemical, and *DO NOT* apply ointments or creams to the burn area.

•Seek medical care.

IF THE VICTIM IS HAVING BREATHING DIFFICULTIES OR LOSES CONSCIOUSNESS

•Check the victim's ABCs and treat as necessary (see page 9).

•Call 911 (EMS).

•To help prevent shock, lay the victim down with legs elevated (this will increase blood flow to the heart and brain) and keep him warm with a blanket or coat (see page 147). The shock position should *NOT* be used if the victim is having difficulty breathing. *AVOID* moving the victim if a spinal cord injury is suspected (see page 154).

CHECK

AIRWAY

BREATHING

CIRCULATION

•If you can, tell EMS what chemical has burned the victim.

CHEMICAL POISONING

See Poisoning and Drug Overdose, page 131

CHEST PAIN

If a victim complains of chest pain, it could mean many things. He may be suffering from a heart problem, such as a heart attack (acute myocardial infarction, see page 111) or angina (chest pain due to lack of oxygen to the heart). The victim may have sustained a chest injury, or he may have a condition such as pleurisy (inflammation of the lung tissue). Sometimes the cause is minor, such as stomach irritation or heartburn.

It isn't always easy (even for medical personnel) to distinguish between a heart problem and another, less serious problem. Chest pain should always be taken seriously, so be sure to seek immediate medical attention.

You should always make sure to call 911 (EMS) immediately if

•Chest pain is sudden or severe or does not subside
•Chest pain spreads to the victim's back, neck, jaw, left shoulder, or arm
•The victim has heart disease
•Chest pain worsens with exercise or exertion
•The victim feels faint or is losing consciousness
•Chest pain is accompanied by shortness of breath, nausea, or vomiting

CHILD ABUSE

Child abuse can take several forms—physical, emotional, and sexual. Certain signs (page 61) may indicate which type of abuse is present. But be aware that there may be a lot of overlap between types of abuse.

All types of abuse will damage a child in countless ways, sometimes for life. That's why decisive action is vital. By confronting the issue, taking charge, and involving the proper authorities, you can help stop the abuse and protect the child now and in the future.

What To Look For

PHYSICAL ABUSE
•Unexplained bruising, marks, burns, broken bones, or cuts
•Torn clothes or untidy appearance
•Extreme fear of parents or other adults
•Unusual behavior—overly aggressive or withdrawn
•Frequent medical care for unexplained injuries

SEXUAL ABUSE
•Discomfort, bruising, and bleeding in the genital area
•Pain when urinating
•Difficulty when sitting or walking
•Sexually transmitted disease
•Pregnancy
•Extreme fear of a person or place
•Abrupt change in behavior
•Tries too hard to please parents or other adults
•Sudden awareness of genitals and sexual acts
•Drawings that depict sexual acts

EMOTIONAL ABUSE
•Infantile behavior—sucking thumb, rocking
•Falls behind at school
•Speech difficulties
•Problems with sleeping or playing
•Antisocial or aggressive behavior
•Withdrawal from life and people
•Attempted suicide

CHECK

AIRWAY

BREATHING

CIRCULATION

What To Do (and Not To Do)

IF THE CHILD IS PHYSICALLY INJURED OR UNCONSCIOUS

•Check the child's ABCs and treat as necessary (see page 9).

•Call 911 (EMS).

•Attend to any physical injuries.

•To help prevent shock, lay the child down with legs elevated (this will increase blood flow to the heart and brain) and keep him warm with a blanket or coat (see page 147). *AVOID* moving the child if a spinal cord injury is suspected (see page 154).

•Calm the child and wait with him until EMS arrive.

OTHER STEPS TO TAKE

•Comfort the child and let him know that you can be trusted.

•Encourage the child to tell you about the abuse.

•Listen carefully to the child and take him seriously.

•Report the abuse. You can talk to a doctor, teacher, police officer, counselor, or child protection worker.

•Ask about support and counseling services.

CHILDBIRTH (EMERGENCY DELIVERY)

Labor normally lasts several hours, so there is usually plenty of time for an expectant mother to get to the hospital or, if prearranged, for a midwife or doctor to get to her home.

Still, labor can happen more quickly for mothers who have given birth previously or who have had quick deliveries before. In the case of premature labor, delivery can also occur unexpectedly. In these cases, there may not be time to get to the hospital, and you may have to deliver the baby or, at least, help out until EMS arrive.

What To Look For

•A previous pregnancy or labor that was rapid

•Water has broken (amniotic sac is ruptured)

•Contractions are less than 2 minutes apart and last 45 to 60 seconds

•Feeling that a bowel movement is coming

•Strong desire to push

•Baby's head is visible at vaginal opening

What To Do (and Not To Do)

•Call 911 (EMS).

•Reassure the mother; point out that most deliveries take place without any complications.

•Quickly gather the supplies you will need (see Supplies for Emergency Childbirth).

•Wash your hands with soap and water. Put on sterile latex gloves if you have them.

•Find a well-lit area that has a large, flat, sturdy surface, such as a bed or table. If nothing else is available, a clean area on the ground or floor will be sufficient.

•Put down plastic sheeting or newspaper, and cover it with clean sheets or other material.

•Place the mother on her back with her knees bent and legs spread. Elevate her hips with towels. Other positions may be more comfortable for her, such as squatting, lying on her left side, or kneeling.

•Remove the mother's underpants and push clothing up to her waist. If she's wearing pants, take them off too.

•Comfort the mother and encourage her to take short, rapid breaths during contractions. During labor, she may vomit or have a bowel movement. So keep a container, such as a pail or pot, and a damp cloth nearby.

•*DO NOT* try to slow the labor by closing her legs.

•In a normal birth, the head will deliver first. If the baby's feet or buttocks or the umbilical cord appear first, see Childbirth Problems, page 66.

•When you see the head, support it with one hand while it delivers, thus preventing the baby from emerging too quickly. *DO NOT* push on the two soft spots (fontanels). They are located near the brow at the front of the head and near the back of the head.

SUPPLIES FOR EMERGENCY CHILDBIRTH

•Plenty of clean sheets, towels, and blankets

•Pillows

•Plastic sheeting or newspaper

•Clean latex gloves

•Sterile gauze dressings

•Rubber suction bulb

•Infant blanket

•Sanitary pads

•Sterile scissors or knife; if you do not have time or are unable to sterilize these items, clean them in soapy water

•Thick string or shoelaces

•Plastic bags

•Container, such as a pail or pot, to catch vomit

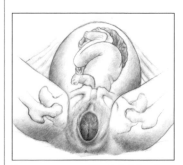

First appearance of the baby's head.

•If the baby's head is still enclosed in the amniotic sac, gently tear the sac open with your fingers, and clear it away from the baby's head and mouth.

•When the head is delivered, use your index finger to check if the umbilical cord is wrapped around the baby's neck. If it is, try to slip it over the baby's head or shoulder. If you can't remove it, clamp and cut the cord immediately, using the following procedure (to cut a cord that is not wrapped around a baby's neck, see page 65):

> •Use new shoelaces or two pieces of thick string. *AVOID* using thread.
>
> •Tie off the cord in two places, with the ties about 2 to 4 inches apart; make the ties on the cord where the cord is around the neck and make each knot tight.
>
> •Using a sterile (or clean) scissors or knife, carefully cut the cord between the two ties; the cord will then unravel from the neck.
>
> •Don't worry about hurting the mother or child—they won't feel any pain when the umbilical cord is cut.

•Wipe fluid from the baby's mouth and nose using sterile gauze or suction. Ask the mother *not* to push while you do this.

•Support the baby with both hands as the rest of the body emerges.

•When you see the feet, grasp them, keeping the baby level with the mother's vagina.

•Dry the baby. Then, using sterile gauze, wipe the baby's mouth and nose. If possible, suction them out as well.

•Usually, the baby will begin breathing on his own. If not, rub his back, or flick your index finger against the soles of the feet. *DO NOT* hold the baby up by his feet and slap his buttocks.

•If the baby isn't breathing, provide two rescue breaths immediately (see page 20). Repeat if necessary until the baby is breathing.

•Wrap the baby in a warm blanket and place him

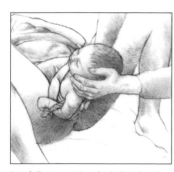

Carefully supporting the baby's head and shoulders as they emerge.

CUTTING THE UMBILICAL CORD

After the baby is delivered, the cord can be left intact, until the mother and child reach the hospital. If medical personnel will not be seen promptly, the cord can be cut at home using the following procedure:

•Use new shoelaces or two pieces of thick string. *AVOID* using thread.

•Tie one string tightly around the cord at least 4 inches away from the baby's navel; tie the other string tightly around the cord 2 to 4 inches away from the first tie, and farther away from the baby.

•Using a sterile (or clean) scissors or knife, carefully cut the cord between the two ties.

•Don't worry about hurting the mother or child—they won't feel any pain when the cord is cut.

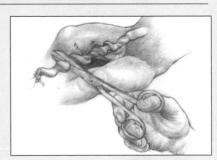

Cutting the umbilical cord after delivery.

To cut a cord that is wrapped around a baby's neck during childbirth, see page 64.

on one side, with the head slightly lower than the rest of the body.

•If the cord is not already cut, it can be left intact (in normal deliveries) until the mother and child reach the hospital. To cut an umbilical cord, see Cutting the Umbilical Cord, above.

•You can give fluids to the mother, but *DO NOT* give her any drinks that contain alcohol.

THE PLACENTA

•It will take about 5 to 30 minutes for the placenta to deliver. If it doesn't deliver within this time, serious bleeding may develop. Immediate medical attention is needed.

•Never pull on the umbilical cord to get the placenta out faster. Gently massaging the uterus (the firm area in the lower abdomen) can help speed up the process and reduce bleeding.

•Once the placenta has delivered, wrap it with the umbilical cord in a towel and place in a plastic bag. Take the placenta to the hospital so the medical personnel can examine it.

•Place a sanitary pad over the mother's vagina to absorb blood. Straighten her legs and help her to hold them together.

CHILDBIRTH PROBLEMS

BREECH BIRTH

Sometimes, the baby's buttocks or legs will appear before the head. This type of delivery can be difficult and should be done by medical personnel, if possible.

•Place the mother with her head down and buttocks up. This will reduce pressure in the birth canal.

•Allow the delivery to progress naturally.

•If the baby's head doesn't emerge within 3 minutes of the rest of the body, the baby is in danger of suffocating. Take the following steps:

  •*DO NOT* try to pull the baby's head out.

  •Put one hand in the mother's vagina, with your palm toward the baby's face.

  •Place your fingers on either side of the nose, and push away the vaginal wall.

  •Encourage the mother to keep pushing. Continue holding the vaginal wall away from the baby, until his head has emerged.

PROLAPSED CORD

If the umbilical cord is delivered before the baby, it may be squeezed during delivery, cutting off the baby's oxygen supply.

•Place the mother with her head down and buttocks up. This will reduce pressure in the birth canal.

•Put one hand into the vagina, and hold the cord away from the baby's body. *DO NOT* try to push the cord back in.

•If EMS haven't arrived, take the mother to the hospital immediately, continuing to hold the cord away from the baby's body. A cesarean section (where the baby is delivered through the abdomen by surgery) may be needed.

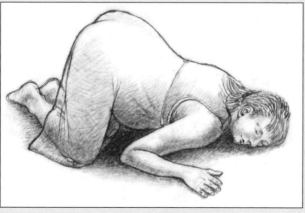

Position for the mother who is having a breech birth or who has a prolapsed cord.

CHOKING

Choking occurs when an object gets stuck in the throat and partly or completely blocks the airway. Breathing becomes difficult or even impossible. Adults commonly choke on food, while young children often choke on small toys, marbles, or coins.

How you help a choking victim depends on the age of the victim, whether he is conscious, and if the victim is pregnant or obese. There is much you can do to provide aid to a choking victim to dislodge a foreign object from the victim's airway, including using abdominal thrusts (the Heimlich maneuver), chest thrusts, and back blows.

What To Look For

- Difficulty speaking
- Difficulty breathing
- Panic
- Grasping or pointing to the throat
- Coughing
- Red face that can later turn blue
- Convulsions
- Loss of consciousness

What To Do (and Not To Do)

ADULTS AND CHILDREN (OVER 1 YEAR OF AGE)

Conscious Victim

IF THE VICTIM CAN TALK, COUGHS EFFECTIVELY, AND APPEARS TO BE MAKING GOOD BREATHING EFFORTS

- Encourage him to cough to try and get rid of the object. *DO NOT* help the victim get rid of the object by, for instance, slapping him on the back.
- *DO NOT* use abdominal or chest thrusts.

PREVENTION POINTERS

To prevent choking in young children, keep small objects, including coins and small toys, away from them, and do not give young children nuts, whole grapes, whole or large pieces of hot dogs, thickly spread peanut butter, or other "chokeable" foods to eat. Taking a first aid basic life support course is also a good idea (see page 178 for more child safety tips).

IF THE VICTIM CAN'T TALK, AND HAS A WEAK COUGH OR BREATHING DIFFICULTIES
•Give 5 abdominal thrusts (see Abdominal Thrusts, page 69).
•If the victim is pregnant or obese, use 5 chest thrusts instead (see Chest Thrusts, page 70).
•Repeat the thrusts until the object is dislodged or the victim loses consciousness (see below).

Unconscious Victim
•Send someone to call 911 (EMS). If you are alone, call EMS after attending to the victim.
•Open the victim's airway:
  •Place one hand on the victim's forehead and gently tilt it backward.
  •Put the other hand under the bony part of the chin and lift, keeping the victim's mouth open.
  •If you suspect a spinal injury, *DO NOT* move the victim's head or neck. Try lifting the chin without tilting the victim's head back (for more details, see page 155).
  •Check the victim's breathing by watching his chest rise and fall. Listen for air coming from the victim's mouth and nose.
•If the victim is not breathing:
  •Keep the head tilted and chin lifted as above.
  •Pinch the nose shut.
  •Give 2 slow rescue breaths. Give enough air so that the victim's chest rises. Allow the chest to fall before giving the next breath.
•If the victim's chest is not rising and breaths are not going in:
  •Give 5 abdominal thrusts (see Abdominal Thrusts, page 69).
  •If the victim is pregnant or obese, use 5 chest thrusts instead (see Chest Thrusts, page 70).
  •Check the mouth and try to dislodge the object. With one hand, grasp the victim's tongue and jaw and lift the jaw. Slide the index finger of your other hand down the inside of the cheek

RESCUE MANEUVERS

ABDOMINAL THRUSTS (HEIMLICH MANEUVER; FOR ADULTS AND CHILDREN OVER 1 YEAR OF AGE)

CONSCIOUS VICTIM
•Stand behind the victim and wrap your arms around his waist, without touching the ribs.
•With one hand, make a fist and put the thumb side just above the navel and well below the breastbone—about the middle of the abdomen.
•Grip the fist with your other hand.
•Keeping your elbows pointing out, give 5 thrusts, pressing your fist inward with a quick, upward motion. Each thrust is meant to dislodge the object and should be done firmly and separately.

UNCONSCIOUS VICTIM
•Put the victim on his back.
•Straddle the victim's thighs.
•Place the heel of one hand just above the navel and well below the breastbone—about the middle of the abdomen.
•Put the other hand on top. Fingers should be pointing towards the victim's head.
•Press inward and upward with 5 quick thrusts.
•Each thrust is meant to dislodge the object and should be done firmly and separately.

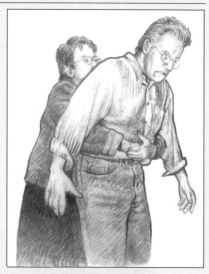

Abdominal thrust (Heimlich maneuver) for a conscious adult or child over 1 year of age.

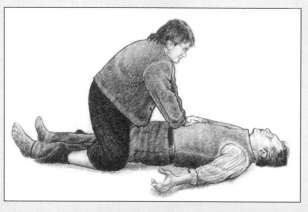

Abdominal thrust (Heimlich maneuver) for an unconscious adult or child over 1 year of age.

(continued)

RESCUE MANEUVERS *(continued)*

CHEST THRUSTS (FOR PREGNANT OR OBESE VICTIMS)

CONSCIOUS VICTIM

•Stand behind the victim and wrap your arms under the victim's armpits.

•Place a fist in the middle of the victim's breastbone at an imaginary line that runs between the nipples.

•Grip the fist with your other hand.

•Keeping your elbows pointing out, give 5 chest thrusts, pressing your fist inward with a quick, upward motion. Each thrust is meant to dislodge the object and should be done firmly and separately.

UNCONSCIOUS VICTIM

•Place the victim on his back. *DO NOT* straddle the victim. Work from the side instead, placing yourself at right angles to the victim.

•Place the heel of one hand on the center of the breastbone in the middle of an imaginary nipple line.

•Put your other hand on top and intertwine your fingers.

•Position your body over your hands, with your arms straight and elbows locked.

•Give 5 firm thrusts. Each thrust is meant to dislodge the object and should be done firmly and separately.

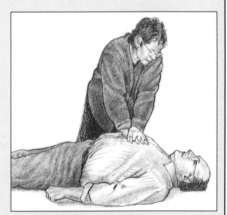

Chest thrust for an unconscious obese person or a pregnant victim.

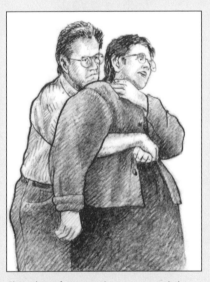

Chest thrust for a conscious pregnant victim or someone who is obese .

and deep into the mouth. If you feel the object, grab it with your finger and remove it. *Be careful not to push it in more deeply.*

•If you can't dislodge the object, give 1 rescue breath, 5 abdominal (or chest) thrusts, and check the mouth. Repeat these steps until the object is dislodged and the victim is breathing or until EMS arrive.

BABIES (NEWBORN TO 1 YEAR OF AGE)

Conscious Baby

IF THE BABY HAS A STRONG COUGH, CRIES, AND APPEARS TO BE MAKING GOOD BREATHING EFFORTS

•Place the baby in a sitting position.

•*DO NOT* interfere with the baby's coughing. *DO NOT* help by, for instance, slapping the baby on the back.

IF THE BABY HAS A WEAK COUGH, BLUE LIPS, BREATHING DIFFICULTIES, AND CAN'T CRY

•Give 5 back blows (see Back Blows for Babies, page 72).

•Give 5 chest thrusts (see Chest Thrusts for Babies, page 72).

•Alternate 5 back blows with 5 chest thrusts until the object is dislodged or the baby loses consciousness (see below).

Unconscious Baby

•Send someone to call 911 (EMS). If you are alone, call EMS after attending to the baby.

•Place the baby on his back.

•Open the airway:

 •Place one hand on the baby's forehead and gently tilt it back slightly.

 •Put the index finger of your other hand under the bony part of the chin and lift, keeping the baby's mouth open. If you suspect a spinal cord injury, don't lift or move the baby's

RESCUE MANEUVERS FOR BABIES

BACK BLOWS FOR BABIES (UNDER 1 YEAR OF AGE)

•Rest your forearm on your thigh. Place the baby face down on your straight forearm with the head lower than the body.

•With one hand, hold the baby's jaw between your thumb and index finger.

•With the heel of your other hand, provide 5 blows between the baby's shoulder blades. Each thrust is meant to dislodge the object and should be done firmly and separately.

CHEST THRUSTS FOR BABIES (UNDER 1 YEAR OF AGE)

•Rest your forearm on your thigh. Place the baby face up on your straight forearm with the head lower than the body.

•Use one hand to support the baby's head and neck.

•Place the middle and index fingers of your other hand on the baby's breastbone just below the nipples.

•Give 5 separate and distinct chest thrusts, pushing in $1/2$ to 1 inch. Keep your fingers on the baby's chest between thrusts.

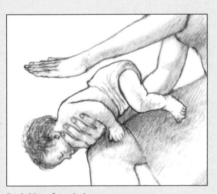

Back blow for a baby.

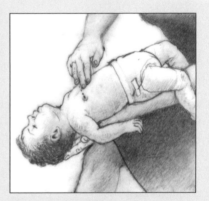

Chest thrust for a baby.

head or neck. Try lifting the chin without tilting the head.

•Check the baby's breathing by watching the chest rise and fall, listening for air from the mouth and nose, and feeling for air against your cheek.

•If the baby is not breathing:

•Keep the head tilted and chin lifted (as above).

•Cover the baby's mouth and nose with your mouth.

•Give 2 slow rescue breaths. Give enough air so that the baby's chest rises. Allow the chest to fall before giving another breath.

•If the baby's chest is not rising and breaths are not going in:

> •Give back blows (see Back Blows for Babies, page 72).
>
> •Give chest thrusts (see Chest Thrusts for Babies, page 72).
>
> •Check the baby's mouth and try to dislodge the object. With one hand, grasp the baby's tongue and jaw between your thumb and fingers, and lift the jaw. If you can see the object, remove it by sliding the index finger of your other hand down the inside of the cheek to the base of the tongue. *DO NOT* try to remove an object you can't see. *Be careful not to push the object in more deeply.*
>
> •Continue with 1 rescue breath followed by 5 back blows and 5 chest thrusts until the object is dislodged or EMS arrive.

COLD EXPOSURE

When exposed to cold temperatures, the body is susceptible to injuries such as frostbite (see page 102) and hypothermia (see page 117).

Frostbite is a condition in which layers of skin and flesh freeze due to temperatures dropping below the freezing mark. Feet, hands, ears, and the nose are most often affected by frostbite. Untreated, frostbite can lead to skin damage and even loss of limbs, toes, and fingers.

With hypothermia, the body can't produce heat as quickly as it loses it. As a result, the body's internal temperature drops below 95°F. Hypothermia can be brought on by below-freezing temperatures, but it can also develop in warm environments. Hypothermia is a serious condition that can be life-threatening.

Fortunately, first aid measures can be performed in wild, remote locations or closer to home, to help prevent or minimize damage from cold exposure.

CPR

See page 12

CUTS (LACERATIONS)

A cut is a break in the skin that can cause external bleeding and possibly infection. A cut can be smooth (caused by a knife, for instance) or jagged (caused by a rough object such as barbed wire).

You can easily treat minor cuts with simple measures at home. Severe cuts may require stitches and emergency medical treatment.

What To Look For
•Cut in the skin
•Bleeding from the cut
•Rapid, weak pulse
•Pale, cold, clammy skin
•Sweating

What To Do (and Not To Do)
•Wash your hands with soap and water. Use gloves if available.
•Remove or cut away any of the victim's clothing covering the wound, as well as any rings and constricting jewelry.

IF THE CUT AND BLEEDING ARE NOT SEVERE
•Wash the wound with soap and water, removing all dirt and debris.
•Exert direct pressure to stop the bleeding.
•Apply antibiotic cream and cover with a clean, dry dressing. *DO NOT* use iodine solutions on the wound; these solutions can hurt already injured tissues and can produce an allergic reaction in some people.
•If the cut's edges are gaping open, hold the edges together and secure with a butterfly bandage or adhesive tape.

•Keep an eye on the cut. If signs of infection appear (pain, swelling, fever, or red streaks), seek medical care.

IF THE CUT IS DEEP AND THE BLEEDING SEVERE

•Check the victim's ABCs and treat as necessary (see page 9)

•Call 911 (EMS).

•To help prevent shock, lay the victim down with legs elevated (this will increase blood flow to the heart and brain) and keep him warm with a blanket or coat (see page 147). *AVOID* moving a victim if a spinal cord injury is suspected (see page 154).

•Control the bleeding by placing a sterile pad or clean cloth over the wound and applying direct, constant pressure. *DO NOT* wash wounds that are deep and bleeding severely since this might increase or restart the bleeding. *DO NOT* remove blood-stained dressings; instead, place another on top to soak up the blood.

•If an embedded object or a protruding bone is present, *DO NOT* apply direct pressure and *DO NOT* remove the embedded object; press down firmly on either side of the injury. Also, direct pressure should never be used for treating eye injuries (see page 92) or head injuries in which a skull fracture is suspected (see page 107).

•If bleeding doesn't stop, apply harder pressure with both hands over a greater area.

•If possible, elevate the wound above the victim's heart level, while still maintaining the pressure.

•If the bleeding continues, apply pressure at the victim's pressure points (where a blood vessel is near the skin's surface and close to a bone). This will limit blood flow to the injury. There are two major pressure points:

  •The *femoral artery* in the groin, where the lower abdomen meets the inner part of the thigh (use for a leg injury): Feel for a pulse in the groin. Then, using your fingers and with your arm extended straight, press the artery

CHECK
_____

Airway
Breathing
Circulation

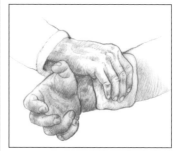
Applying direct pressure to a wound.

against the pelvic bone until you can't feel a pulse. Use both hands if necessary.

•The *brachial artery* on the upper inside arm (use for arm injuries): You can find it by feeling for a pulse below the round muscle of the biceps, halfway between the armpit and elbow. Using your fingers, press the artery until you can't feel a pulse.

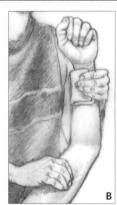

Location of major pressure points. (A) If bleeding from a leg wound cannot be stopped by direct compression and elevation, the femoral artery in the groin can be compressed to limit blood flow to the leg. (B) Likewise, the brachial artery in the upper arm, between the armpit and elbow, can be compressed to limit blood flow to the rest of the arm.

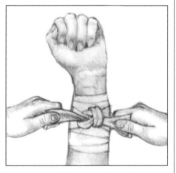

Applying a pressure bandage.

•After the bleeding stops, apply a pressure bandage. While pulling steadily, wrap a roller gauze bandage or long cloth tightly over the dressing, and above and below the wound. Split the bandage end into two strips, then knot the ends tightly, directly over the wound. A pressure bandage should be tight enough to keep pressure on the wound but not so tight that it cuts off circulation. A bandage is too tight if there is no pulse beyond the wound (away from the victim's trunk) or the skin in that area is turning blue.

•In general, a tourniquet (a strip of material placed tightly around a limb to stop the flow of blood) is *NOT* recommended, as it might damage nerves and blood vessels.

•Calm the victim and stay with him until EMS has arrived.

•Ask about the victim's tetanus immunization status. If it is not up to date, the victim may need a tetanus shot, especially if he was cut by a dirty object.

DEHYDRATION

Dehydration occurs when you lose more fluids than you take in. Profuse sweating (caused by strenuous exercise or a fever) and persistent vomiting or diarrhea can lead to dehydration if you fail to replace the fluids lost. Even cold-weather activities can put you at risk—fluids are lost when the cold air you inhale must be moistened and warmed by your body, and because low temperature causes an increase in urination.

Even under normal conditions, you often need to drink at least 2 quarts of fluid per day to prevent dehydration. That's because you lose this fluid simply by carrying out the basics of life, such as breathing and urinating.

Dehydration, if left untreated, is serious and potentially life-threatening. By knowing the signs of fluid depletion and acting fast to reverse it, you can help a victim avoid any serious consequences of dehydration.

What To Look For
•Dark yellow urine
•Infrequent urination (less than 5 times a day)
•Extreme thirst
•Fatigue
•Muscle or abdominal cramps
•Lightheadedness or dizziness, especially when rising

What To Do (and Not To Do)
•Sit the victim down. If it's a hot day, move him into a shaded, cool area.
•Replace lost fluids by giving the victim plenty of water. Commercial sports drinks (such as Gatorade) can be given. *AVOID* giving drinks containing caffeine, alcohol, or high amounts of sugar, because they increase urination.

PREVENTION POINTERS

Preventing dehydration is a simple task. All you need to do is drink fluids, preferably water, on a regular basis throughout the day—even if you're not thirsty. When you're exercising, be sure to increase your fluid intake before, during, and after your activity. And always drink more than you think you need (see Sports Injuries, page 215).

D–E

PREVENTION POINTERS

Sports and other activities are the source of many dental injuries. Wearing a properly fitted mouthguard when it's required can protect your teeth, braces, or bridgework when the going gets rough. See Sports Injuries, page 215.

D–E

•Get medical help if the signs and symptoms persist or if nausea, vomiting, or seizures occur.

DENTAL PAIN AND INJURIES

Cavities and infections are a common cause of dental pain, although food or objects caught between the teeth can be the cause as well. Dental pain may be limited to one tooth, or it may spread further afield to the face, neck, and jaw. Whenever dental pain arises, whether mild or severe, be sure the victim sees his dentist.

Dental injuries can include a knocked-out tooth (partial or complete), broken or chipped teeth, bites to the tongue or lip, or damaged dental work.

There are steps you can take to improve the outcome of many dental injuries. A knocked-out tooth, for instance, may be reimplanted if you store it properly and seek dental care immediately.

What To Look For

DENTAL PAIN
•Pain in tooth that may extend to the eye, ear, neck, or jaw
•Tooth sensitivity to heat and cold
•Swollen gums around the affected tooth
•Persistent bad breath
•Fever
•Inability to open mouth fully

DENTAL INJURIES
•Evidence of a fall or other injury to the mouth
•Missing tooth
•Tooth hanging by its root
•Bleeding from the mouth or tooth socket
•Difficulty breathing
•Rapid, weak pulse
•Pale, cold, clammy skin
•Sweating
•Skin around the mouth and lips is blue (see also page 15)

What To Do (and Not To Do)

DENTAL PAIN

•If the dental pain is accompanied by fever or inability to open mouth fully, seek dental care immediately.

•Ask the victim to rinse his mouth with warm water.

•Use dental floss to remove any food particles or other objects caught between the victim's teeth. *DO NOT* stick anything on or into the aching tooth.

•Place a covered ice pack or cold compress to the affected side of the face. Alternatively, the victim may find heat from a covered hot water bottle more soothing.

•Give the victim acetaminophen or ibuprofen or, if an adult, aspirin to relieve the pain. The medication should be swallowed with water, *NOT* placed directly on the aching tooth.

•Seek dental care.

DENTAL INJURY

Bite to the tongue or lip

•Ask the victim to rinse his mouth with water.

•Sit the victim down with his head forward to let blood drain into a container. Ask the victim not to swallow.

•To stop the bleeding, apply direct pressure to the wound with a clean gauze pad or cloth.

•To reduce swelling and pain, place an ice pack (wrapped in a cloth) or a cold compress against the victim's face.

•If the wound is large or continues to bleed, seek medical care. Stitches may be needed.

•If the bleeding is severe

•Check the victim's ABCs and treat as necessary (see page 9).

•Call 911 (EMS).

•To help prevent shock, lay the victim down with legs elevated (this will increase blood flow to the heart and brain) and keep him warm with a blanket or coat (see page 147). *AVOID* moving

D-E

CHECK

Airway

Breathing

Circulation

the victim if a spinal cord injury is suspected (see page 154).

•Continue to apply pressure to the wound until EMS arrive.

•*DO NOT* give the victim food or drink.

Broken Tooth

•Have the victim rinse his mouth with water. *DO NOT* give the victim food or drink.

•To reduce swelling and pain, place an ice pack (wrapped in a cloth) or a cold compress against the victim's face.

•Cover the broken tooth with a sterile gauze pad.

•Seek immediate dental care. If the tooth is chipped, it may only need to be filed down. If the break extends down to the tooth's root, more thorough dental care will be required.

Knocked-Out Tooth

•If the tooth is partially knocked out

•Put the tooth back in the socket. *DO NOT* rinse or clean it.

•If the tooth is completely knocked out

•*DO NOT* rinse or clean the tooth unless the tooth is very dirty. If so, gently rinse away large debris.

•If the victim is an adult, place the tooth back in the socket and ask him to hold it in place with a sterile gauze pad. Alternatively, the tooth can be held under the tongue. *DO NOT* use this procedure if the victim is a child or an adult who is unable to cooperate, as he may swallow the tooth by mistake. Instead, place the tooth in a container of the victim's saliva or whole milk (not skim or powdered). *DO NOT* touch the tooth's root.

Take the victim to the dentist immediately.

Broken Dental Work

•If dental work (such as a crown) is broken, leave it in the victim's mouth. If the dental work falls out on its own, keep it to show the dentist.

D–E

DID YOU KNOW...

Many times a knocked-out tooth can be reimplanted if it is properly saved and transported to a dentist.

•Always remove damaged, loose dentures to prevent them from falling into the throat and blocking the airway. If the damaged dentures are not loose, leave them in the victim's mouth. Seek dental care.

DIABETIC EMERGENCIES

Insulin is a hormone that breaks food down into blood sugar, which is used as fuel by the body. People with diabetes don't produce enough insulin or can't use the insulin their body does produce. As a result, it's difficult for them to control their blood sugar (glucose) levels by natural means. Other self-imposed methods, including diet, insulin injections, and oral diabetes medications, are needed to keep glucose levels in check.

But even in people who carefully control their diabetes, emergencies such as low blood sugar (hypoglycemia) or high blood sugar (hyperglycemia) can occur. Low blood sugar may be caused by changes in insulin absorption, changes in activity levels, or changes in eating habits. High blood sugar may be caused by poor diet, missed insulin shots or oral medications, or infections.

Diabetic emergencies can be serious, but most can be prevented or reversed in their early stages. You can do this by recognizing the signs and symptoms—which may appear suddenly or gradually—and treating them promptly.

What To Look For

LOW BLOOD SUGAR (HYPOGLYCEMIA)
•Hunger
•Weakness, dizziness
•Pale, cold, clammy skin
•Sweating
•Rapid or pounding pulse
•Confusion, irritability, aggressiveness
•Poor coordination, staggering
•Headache

FOR MORE INFORMATION...

Organizations such as the American Diabetes Association are good sources of information on diabetes. See page 246.

D–E

DID YOU KNOW...

Low blood sugar is one of the most common causes of a sudden change in mental status.

• Nausea and vomiting
• Seizures
• Loss of consciousness

HIGH BLOOD SUGAR (HYPERGLYCEMIA)

• Extreme thirst
• Frequent urination
• Strange, sweet-smelling breath
• Fatigue, drowsiness
• Weakness
• Loss of appetite
• Headache
• Nausea and vomiting
• Agitation
• Abdominal pain
• Flushed, warm skin
• Seizures
• Loss of consciousness

What To Do (and Not To Do)

UNKNOWN BLOOD SUGAR STATUS

IF THE VICTIM IS UNCONSCIOUS

• Put a small amount of table sugar under his tongue.
• Check the victim's ABCs and treat as necessary (see page 9).
• Call 911 (EMS).
• To help prevent shock, lay the victim down with legs elevated (this will increase blood flow to the heart and brain) and keep him warm with a blanket or coat (see page 147). *AVOID* moving the victim if a spinal cord injury is suspected (for more details, see page 154).

IF THE VICTIM IS CONSCIOUS

• Give the victim food or drink containing sugar (such as juice, a nondiet soft drink, or candy).
• If symptoms don't improve in 10 minutes, call 911 (EMS) and treat as above.

CHECK

AIRWAY
BREATHING
CIRCULATION

D–E

LOW BLOOD SUGAR (HYPOGLYCEMIA)
•Immediately give the victim food or drink containing sugar.
•If symptoms don't go away in 10 minutes, again give food or drink containing sugar.
•A medicine called glucagon raises blood sugar rapidly. If the victim has glucagon, inject it immediately.
•If symptoms still don't go away or the victim doesn't have glucagon, call 911 (EMS).
•Consult a doctor to determine the cause of the hypoglycemia.

HIGH BLOOD SUGAR (HYPERGLYCEMIA)
•Help the victim take his usual insulin dose or oral diabetes medication, if not taken already.
•Give the victim unsweetened fluids.
•If symptoms don't begin to improve, make sure to call 911 (EMS).

DISLOCATIONS

A dislocation is the separation of a bone from a joint. It can occur if a joint is forced, by a blow or fall, into an abnormal position. The joints in the shoulder, thumb, finger, and jaw are those most commonly dislocated. Sometimes dislocations can correct themselves, but most will require emergency medical attention.

It's often hard to tell if an injury is a dislocation or a broken bone. When in doubt, treat it as a broken bone (see page 50).

What To Look For
•Pain, tenderness and swelling at the injury site
•Limb hanging in an unusual position from the victim's joint
•Joint unable to move

What To Do (and Not To Do)
•Check the victim's ABCs and treat as necessary (see page 9).

CHECK

Airway

Breathing

Circulation

D–E

D-E

•Call 911 (EMS).

•If necessary, remove or cut away clothing around the injury.

•If there is bleeding, take steps to control it (see page 38).

•Check for pain, swelling, and tenderness at the injury site. Make every effort not to move the injured area.

•Immobilize the injury by padding it with pillows and towels. If EMS are not nearby and you must transport the victim to the hospital, you may need to splint the dislocation (see page 52).

•Place an ice pack (wrapped in a cloth) or a cold compress on the injured area to ease pain and swelling. If it is not too painful for the victim, elevate the injured part. *DO NOT* try to correct the dislocation, as you may cause further injury.

•To help prevent shock, lay the victim down with legs elevated (this will increase blood flow to the heart and brain) and keep him warm with a blanket or coat (see page 147). *AVOID* moving the victim if a spinal cord injury is suspected (for more details, see page 154).

PREVENTION POINTERS

Water safety should always be observed whether you're around a pool, a pond, or even a puddle. Supervision, personal flotation devices (PFDs), swimming lessons, and avoiding drugs and alcohol before or during water activities are just some of the steps you can take to help prevent a drowning incident. See Safety Around the House and in the Garden (page 195) and Water and Boating Safety (page 212).

DROWNING

Drowning begins as a person struggles to stay afloat in water. As a person attempts to breathe, water may enter both the stomach and the lungs. Eventually, the airway closes, and breathing stops. If the victim is rescued before breathing stops, the event is called near drowning (not drowning).

You can help a victim survive near drowning by knowing its signs and initiating first aid steps.

What To Look For

•Victim may be fully clothed in water

•Panic

•Violent struggle

•Flailing arms

•Sinking body with only the head showing

•Coughing, spluttering
•Loss of consciousness

What To Do (and Not To Do)

•Remove the victim from the water as quickly as possible (see Rescue Techniques, pages 86 and 87).

•In an unconscious victim or in a victim complaining of neck pain, numbness, tingling, or weakness in the arms or legs, assume a spinal cord injury and make every attempt possible to minimize moving the neck (see Spinal Injury, page 154).

•Send someone to call 911 (EMS).

•Remember that hypothermia is always a concern in near-drowning victims; once the victim is on dry land, remove wet clothing and wrap the victim in warm blankets.

RESCUING AN UNCONSCIOUS VICTIM

•Get to the victim as quickly as possible, and turn him face up.

•Rotate the upper half of his body in one motion; try not to twist the head.

•Open the victim's airway and assess the ABCs. Begin rescue breathing if possible, although getting the victim to land and ensuring your own safety are priorities (see page 24).

•Once on land, lay the victim down, and cover him with blankets. Reassess the ABCs and treat as necessary (see page 9). *DO NOT* use abdominal thrusts (Heimlich maneuver) to force water out of the victim.

•*DO NOT* move the victim's head or neck. Try lifting the chin without tilting the head back (see also page 153).

RESCUING A CONSCIOUS VICTIM

•Perform a water or ice rescue (for details, see pages 86 and 87).

•If a spinal cord injury is suspected (neck pain or weakness, numbness, or paralysis in the arms or legs), keep the victim in the water if possible,

CHECK

Airway

Breathing

Circulation

D–E

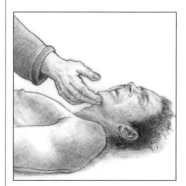

Lifting the victim's chin without tilting the head back.

RESCUE TECHNIQUES

WATER RESCUE

•First, try to reach the victim from the water's edge if possible (unless the victim is in ice water—see page 87) using a long stick, branch, or rope. Ideally, have someone hang onto you while you pull the person out of the water.

•If the person is too far to reach from the water's edge, throw a floatable object, such as a life preserver or inflated spare tire. If a rope is attached, pull the victim out of the water.

•If a row boat is available and you know how to use it, row out to the victim. Throw a floatable object to the victim or have him hold onto the boat while you row back to shore.

•The last resort is to swim to the victim. This should only be done by an experienced rescuer who knows how to control the rescue and not be grabbed and pulled under the water.

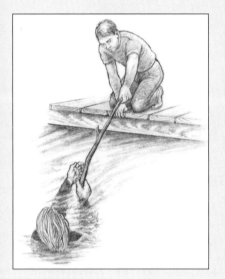

Rescuing the victim from the water's edge when the victim is nearby.

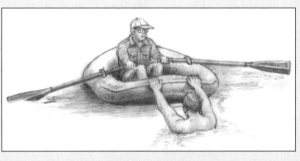

Using a boat to rescue the victim in water.

RESCUE TECHNIQUES *(continued)*

ICE WATER RESCUE
•Have someone call 911 (EMS) while you try to rescue the victim.

•If the victim has fallen through the ice near the shore, stay on the shore and extend a pole, board, or line to the victim and pull him out of the ice and to the shore.

•If you can't reach the victim from shore, lie flat on the ice and push a long object in front of you, such as a pole or ladder, for the victim to grasp. Allow the victim to use the object to pull himself out of the water.

•If other people are present, form a human chain. Some people in the chain should lie on the ice while others should stand on shore ready to pull the chain back.

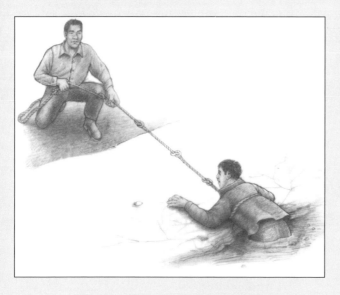

Ice water rescue when the victim is near the shore.

unless the victim is in ice water (see Rescue Techniques, above). Float the head in line with the body, until EMS arrive with a body board to place under the victim and take him to dry land.

•If a spinal cord injury is not suspected, remove the victim from the water, lay him down on coats or a blanket and reassess the ABCs. Turn the victim onto his left side. This is called the recovery position and will allow fluids to drain from his mouth. *DO NOT* use abdominal thrusts (Heimlich maneuver) to force water out of the victim.

•If the victim complains of breathing difficulties, transport him to the nearest medical facility for evaluation.

DRUG OVERDOSE

See Poisoning and Drug Overdose, page 131

PREVENTION POINTERS

Loud noises can damage hearing. An ear protection device, such as ear plugs, should always be used when working or playing in noisy environments.

EARACHE AND EAR INJURY

Ear infections, cold, flu, air travel (see page 200), and earwax blockage are some of the causes of earaches in children and adults. Ear injuries can encompass a whole range of conditions, from cuts on the outer ear to ruptured eardrums. Foreign objects can also get stuck in the ear (see page 99).

In most cases, earaches and ear injuries are not life-threatening. But quick, correct first aid will reduce a victim's pain and help prevent long-term hearing loss.

What To Look For

EARACHE
•Throbbing pain in the ear
•Discharge from the ear
•Difficulty hearing
•Sore throat
•Headache
•Fever
•Dizziness
•Loss of balance

EAR INJURY
•Pain in the ear
•Bleeding from the outer ear or ear canal
•Dizziness
•Nausea and vomiting
•Headache
•Loss of balance
•Difficulty hearing

What To Do (and Not To Do)

EARACHE

•If the victim has severe pain, a high temperature, or discharge from the ear canal, seek immediate medical attention.

•If the ear pain begins suddenly during air travel, try to "pop" the ear by chewing gum, yawning, or swallowing while pinching the nose shut.

•Put the victim in an upright position to reduce pressure and pain in the ear.

•Place a covered hot water bottle on the victim's affected area.

•Give the victim acetaminophen or ibuprofen or, if an adult, aspirin.

•Most cases of earwax blockage can be treated at home, using mineral oil, baby oil, or over-the-counter drops in the blocked ear to soften the wax. Hydrogen peroxide can also help remove it. If your attempts to remove the earwax blockage don't work, see your doctor.

•*DO NOT* put cotton swabs or sharp or pointed objects into the ear canal. They can push the wax further into the ear and cause severe ear damage.

EAR INJURY

•If the victim complains of severe pain from the ear, it could be sign of a ruptured eardrum. Cover the ear with a bandage or cloth and seek immediate medical attention.

•If the victim has a cut (laceration) to the *outside* of the ear, control the bleeding.

IF THE BLEEDING IS NOT SEVERE

•Wash the wound with soap and water.

•Apply direct pressure to stop the bleeding and cover with a clean, dry dressing.

IF THE BLEEDING IS SEVERE

•Check the victim's ABCs and treat as necessary (see page 9)

•Call 911 (EMS).

•Elevate the victim's head.

D–E

CHECK

Airway

Breathing

Circulation

D–E

• Wash your hands with soap and water.

• *DO NOT* remove an object that is embedded in a wound.

• *DO NOT* wash wounds that are deep and bleeding severely, as this could increase or restart the bleeding.

• Place a sterile pad or clean cloth over the wound and apply direct, constant pressure. If bleeding doesn't stop, apply harder pressure with both hands over a greater area. *DO NOT* remove blood-stained dressings. Instead, place another on top to soak up the blood.

IF THE VICTIM HAS BLEEDING OR FLUID COMING FROM *INSIDE* THE EAR CANAL

• Cover the ear with a bandage or cloth, to absorb the blood or fluid. *DO NOT* try to stop the flow of blood or fluid.

• Lay the victim on his injured side, so the blood or fluid can drain out. *AVOID* moving the victim if a head or spinal cord injury is suspected (see Head Injury, page 107, and Spinal Injury, page 154.)

• *DO NOT* stick an object, such as a cotton swab, into the ear.

ELECTRICAL BURNS

A person can be burned if he comes into contact with an electrical current from an outlet, power lines, railways, or even lightning.

There are two main types of electrical burns—arc burns and electrical injury. Arc burns are caused by electricity jumping from one spot to another on the skin. An electrical injury is caused by a current passing through the body. With electrical injuries, burns will appear not only at the site where the current entered the body but also where it came out. Most of the damage, however, is internal, and the injury is sometimes more extensive than was initially apparent.

All electrical burns should be treated as severe. First aid measures can do much to reduce damage

---

PREVENTION POINTERS

You can help prevent electrical burns in your home by playing it safe with electricity. That means installing safety covers on outlets, keeping appliances away from water, and unplugging appliances when they're not in use. And that's just the beginning—see Childproofing Your Home (page 176) and Room-By-Room Safety (page 191). You can also protect yourself and your family from a lightning strike with a few simple measures—see Violent Weather, Lightning (page 218).

to the victim. But be aware that, with electrical burns, you must act carefully to avoid exposing yourself to the electrical current.

What To Look For

•Severe jolt, tingling

•Burn marks on the skin or mouth

•Swelling and charring at points where the current has passed through the body

•Pain

•Headache

•Difficulty breathing

•Muscle or bone pain if the victim was thrown to the ground

•Loss of consciousness

•Heart stops beating (cardiac arrest)

What To Do (and Not To Do)

•Never approach the victim until you're sure the power has been turned off. At home, turn off electricity at the fuse box, circuit breaker, or outside switch box, or unplug the appliance. If the victim has come into contact with high-voltage electricity (such as power lines), call the power company or 911 (EMS) and stay at least 20 feet away until officials have told you it is safe to approach the victim.

•Check the victim's ABCs and treat as necessary (see page 9).

•Cover the burn with clean, non-fluffy material. *DO NOT* apply ointments or creams.

•To help prevent shock, lay the victim down with legs elevated (this will increase blood flow to the heart and brain) and keep him warm with a blanket or coat (see page 147). *AVOID* moving the victim if a spinal cord injury is suspected (for more details, see page 154).

•Seek medical attention if electricity went through the victim's body (for example, in one hand and out the leg), or if there is damage to the skin (this can occur, for instance, when a child chews on an electrical cord).

D–E

CHECK

Airway

Breathing

Circulation

PREVENTION POINTERS

The eyes can be damaged by the sun just as the skin can. Always wear sunglasses that block out 99% to 100% UVA and UVB radiation when you are in the sun.

EYE PROBLEMS OR SUDDEN CHANGE IN VISION

The eye is a sensitive organ that can be easily damaged by blows, burns, or foreign objects (see also page 99). Diseases, such as acute glaucoma, can affect the eyes without warning and impair vision. Inflammation, such as conjunctivitis, can be caused by infection, allergy, medical conditions, or injury.

By providing first aid for eye injuries and vision problems, you can help prevent vision loss in the victim.

What To Look For

EYE INJURY
- Eye pain or severe stinging
- Swelling, bruising, or redness in the eye area
- Bleeding from the eye or eyelid
- Unable to open the eyes
- Tearing
- Rapid blinking
- Dryness, itchiness
- Reduced or double vision or loss of sight

SUDDEN CHANGE IN VISION
- Sudden eye pain and vision changes not related to an injury
- Headache
- Nausea and vomiting
- Reduced or double vision or loss of sight

RED EYE
- Redness of white of the eye
- Change in vision
- Pain with eye movement
- Headache
- Nausea and vomiting
- Discharge from eye or crusting

What To Do (and Not To Do)

•To treat all injuries or sudden changes in vision, remove contact lenses if worn by the victim. Contact lenses can be removed by

>•Holding the victim's upper eyelid open, using your thumb or fingers

>•Sliding the contact lens towards the outer edge of the eye with the thumb of your other hand

>•Pulling the skin at this edge out and down— the lens should come out

>•If you have trouble removing the contact lens, wait for medical personnel to do it.

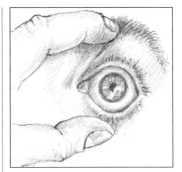

Holding the victim's eyelid open.

EYE INJURIES

Black Eye

•Sit the victim down.

•Apply an ice pack, wrapped in cloth, to reduce pain and swelling. *DO NOT* apply pressure to the injured eye or eye area.

•Seek immediate medical care if

>•Pain, bruising, or swelling is severe or continues

>•Victim's vision is reduced

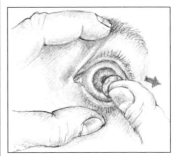

Removing a contact lens from the victim's eye.

Chemical Burns

•Hold the eyelid open and use a gentle stream of water to flush out the chemical for at least 20 minutes. Turn the victim's head so that water does not drain into the uninjured eye. *DO NOT* use an eyecup or eyedrops, unless a doctor or EMS tell you to do so.

•Flush the eye from the nose side to the outside.

•Be sure not to flush the chemical into the victim's other eye.

•Apply dressing and loose bandages to both eyes.

•Get immediate medical care.

Cuts

•Cover both eyes with a dressing and loose bandages, and seek medical attention. *DO NOT* flush

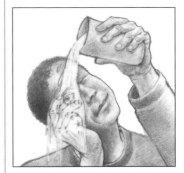

Flushing the eye for a chemical burn.

the eyes and *DO NOT* try to stop the bleeding with direct pressure.

•If the cut and bleeding is severe

   •Call 911 (EMS).

   •To help prevent shock, lay the victim down with legs elevated (this will increase blood flow to the heart and brain) and keep him warm with a blanket or coat (see page 147). *AVOID* moving the victim if a spinal cord injury is suspected (see page 154).

Penetrating Injury

•Call 911 (EMS).

•Lay the victim down.

•Place a paper cup or a cardboard cone over the injured eye, to protect the eye and hold the penetrating object in place. Make sure the cup or cone is larger than the penetrating object. Tape the cup or cone to the victim's face, and secure with bandages wrapped lightly around the head. *DO NOT* flush the eye or attempt to remove an object, such as a needle or knife.

•Cover the uninjured eye with a patch or sterile dressing. This will stop the injured eye from moving around.

•Comfort the victim, and wait with him until EMS arrive.

SUDDEN CHANGE IN VISION

•Calm the victim.

•Seek medical care right away. Surgery may be needed immediately to correct the problem.

RED EYE

•Seek medical care.

•Apply warm compresses.

•Wash the eyelid with nonirritating baby shampoo and rinse the lid well.

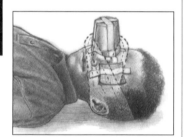

Using a cup to cover an eye with a penetrating injury, a dressing on the uninjured eye, and a bandage (shown with dashed line) to secure the cup and dressing in place.

D–E

FAINTING

Fainting is a sudden, brief loss of consciousness that occurs when the supply of blood to the brain is interrupted. It is often caused by pain, lack of food, emotional upset, or standing too long in one place. Sometimes fainting signals a more serious problem, such as dehydration (not enough fluid in the body, see page 77), bleeding, or heart problems.

By recognizing its signs, you can help prevent fainting and the injuries that can occur when a victim falls.

What To Look For

•Brief loss of consciousness
•Slow pulse, rapid pulse, or palpitations
•Pale, cold, clammy skin
•Sweating
•Dizziness
•Weakness
•Nausea and vomiting
•Blurred vision

What To Do (and Not To Do)

•If possible, try to prevent the victim from falling.
•Lay the victim down, and then elevate and support his feet.
•Turn the victim on his left side—this is called the recovery position (see page 11). It will help prevent further vomiting and allow fluids to drain from his mouth.
•Loosen any tight clothing.
•Open a window or door, to let in fresh air.
•Check the victim for any injuries that may have occurred during the fall.
•Place a cold compress on the victim's forehead.
•As the victim recovers, help him sit up slowly.
•Once you're sure the victim has recovered and can swallow, give him a cold drink containing sugar.

F–H

•You should seek medical attention if the victim
- •Is elderly
- •Has frequent fainting spells
- •Faints for no reason
- •Faints while sitting or lying down
- •Has a history of heart problems

•If the victim doesn't regain consciousness immediately after fainting
- •Check the victim's ABCs and treat as necessary (see page 9).
- •Call 911 (EMS).

CHECK

Airway
Breathing
Circulation

DEHYDRATION AND FEVER

It's important to drink lots of fluids during a fever to prevent dehydration. See page 77.

FEVER

A fever is an increase above normal body temperature. Many things can cause this increase, including colds, sore throats, and middle ear infections. A fever, in fact, is a sign that the body is fighting the illness, whatever it may be.

A fever can be frightening, especially to new parents, but it is often harmless and can be treated with over-the-counter medication and other simple first aid measures.

What To Look For
•Temperature of, or higher than, 100.4°F (if taken by the mouth or in the armpit) or 101.4°F (if taken by the rectum)
•Flushed face
•Sore throat
•Earache
•Hot forehead
•Sweating or chills
•Irritability
•Loss of appetite
•Pale skin
•Headache
•Dry mouth

•Nausea and vomiting

•Diarrhea

•Rapid pulse

What To Do (and Not To Do)

•Give acetaminophen or ibuprofen to a child. If an adult has a fever, aspirin may be used. Aspirin should never be given to a child, unless instructed by a doctor, as it could cause a serious disease called Reye's syndrome.

•Read the medication labels carefully and give as instructed. If in doubt, ask your pharmacist or doctor.

•Give the victim plenty of cool, clear liquids. *DO NOT* force him to eat.

•Dress the victim in lightweight cool clothes so that body heat can escape. *DO NOT* overheat the room.

•Keep the victim quiet. Activity can raise the temperature even more.

•Lukewarm sponge baths may help lower an extremely high fever. Never use cold water or alcohol.

•Call 911 (EMS) or go to the emergency room if the victim

  •Is less than 4 weeks old

  •Has breathing difficulties

  •Has repeated convulsions associated with the fever (febrile convulsions)

  •Has a stiff neck

  •Has a significant change in behavior or mental status

  •Has abdominal pain

  •Has a severe headache

•Call the doctor if

  •The fever lasts longer than 24 hours or if you're anxious about the victim's appearance or behavior

  •Has a new rash

  •Has vomiting and diarrhea for more than a day

  •Has other serious illnesses (such as leukemia)

  •Has difficulty swallowing

F–H

PREVENTION POINTERS

Preventing food poisoning is a simple matter of handling, storing, and cooking food in the proper way. Washing your hands before handling food, refrigerating cooked leftovers within 2 hours, and cooking meat and poultry thoroughly are just some of the ways you can keep food "friendly" (for more details, see Preventing Poisonings, page 186).

FOOD POISONING

Food poisoning is not an allergy, but a reaction to contaminated or spoiled foods. Many types of food, such as undercooked meat and poultry, contaminated or improperly stored shellfish or dairy foods, or cooked food left at room temperature for too long can cause food poisoning.

The signs of food poisoning may appear within a few hours or 24 hours or longer after eating contaminated or spoiled food. Usually, food poisoning is mild and will clear up on its own, although more severe forms, such as botulism, require emergency medical treatment.

What To Look For
- Nausea and vomiting
- Diarrhea
- More than one person affected
- Chills
- Fever
- Abdominal pain and cramping
- Headache
- Dizziness
- Difficulty breathing
- Rash
- Slurred speech
- Double vision
- Loss of consciousness

What To Do (and Not To Do)
- Have the victim rest. Give him plenty of clear fluids. Water, a commercial sports drink (such as Gatorade), or a clear, noncaffeinated soda (such as ginger ale) are good choices. *DO NOT* give the victim dairy products, such as milk. *AVOID* giving the victim any medications to stop the diarrhea or vomiting unless instructed by a doctor.
- Vomiting can happen at any time, so keep a container, such as a pail or pot, and a damp cloth nearby.

•Lay the victim on his left side—this is called the recovery position (see page 11). It will help prevent further vomiting and allow fluids to drain from his mouth.

•If fever persists longer than 24 hours or if the victim can't keep fluids down, call the doctor. (See Dehydration, page 77.)

•If symptoms are severe or don't subside, or if you notice the signs of botulism (slurred speech, dizziness, double vision, difficulty breathing, or loss of consciousness)

  •Check the victim's ABCs and treat as necessary (see page 9).

  •Immediately call 911 (EMS) or your doctor.

  •To help prevent shock, lay the victim down with legs elevated (this will increase blood flow to the heart and brain) and keep him warm with a blanket or coat (see page 147).

FOREIGN OBJECTS IN THE EYE, EAR, NOSE, OR THROAT

Foreign objects, such as eyelashes, insects, dirt, food, and small toys, can get stuck in the eye, ear, nose, or throat. This most often occurs with young children, who tend to push objects into their noses and ears. Swallowing objects is common in this age group as well.

In most cases, an object can easily be removed at home, although foreign bodies, especially in the throat, can sometimes create an emergency situation. You can be prepared by knowing what to do—and what not to do—when a foreign object finds its way into the body.

What To Look For

EYE
•Pain or redness in the eye
•Tearing
•Blurred vision
•Eye rubbed continually

CHECK

Airway

Breathing

Circulation

F–H

PREVENTION POINTERS

How can you prevent your young child from swallowing foreign objects or from pushing objects—including food—into his eyes, ears, or nose? By keeping objects that could cause problems well out of his way. Start by storing buttons, pins, and food in a safe place. And when you're buying toys, make sure they're large and well made (see Childproofing Your Home, page 176).

EAR
- Ear pain
- Difficulty hearing
- Buzzing or movement felt in the ear

NOSE
- Nose runs from one side
- Nose picked continually
- Difficulty breathing through nose
- Foul odor from nose

THROAT
- Difficulty speaking
- Difficulty breathing
- Panic
- Grasping or pointing to the throat
- Coughing
- Red face that later turns blue
- Convulsions
- Loss of consciousness

What To Do (and Not To Do)

EYE
- Tell the victim not to rub his eye.
- Wash your hands with soap and water.
- *DO NOT* try to remove an object that is embedded in the eye (see page 94).
- Ask the victim to sit down facing the light.
- Check under the lower lid first. Pull it down and ask the victim to look up. If you see the object, remove it gently with a cotton swab. *AVOID* poking the eye. You can also flush it out with warm water—have the victim tilt his head so the injured eye is down. Rinse from the inside corner to the outer corner.
- If the object is not under the lower lid, lift the upper lid. If you see it, remove the object as outlined above.

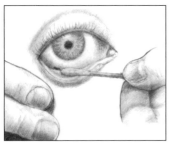

Using a cotton swab to remove a foreign object from the eye.

•Cover the eyes with sunglasses or loose dressing and seek medical help if

•You can't see the object.

•You remove the object but the victim's symptoms remain. You may have only removed part of it, or the cornea may have been scratched.

EAR

An Insect

•Ask the victim to sit down with the affected area facing up.

•See if the insect will crawl out.

•Shine a light into the ear. Some insects will move toward the light and out of the ear. Others, unfortunately, will move away from the light, and the victim will feel more pain. If that's the case, turn the light off immediately.

•If the insect hasn't come out of the ear, gently pour a teaspoon of oil at room temperature (cooking oil, mineral oil, or baby oil) into the victim's ear canal to drown the insect. *DO NOT* pour oil into a child's ear if he has had ear tubes placed in his ears.

•If you can't remove the insect, seek medical help. *DO NOT* try to remove an insect with tweezers or cotton swabs; this may cause it to crawl farther into the ear canal.

Another Object

•If the victim is an adult or an older cooperative child, turn his head so the affected ear is facing down, and remove the object with tweezers. Seek medical care to ensure that the entire object is gone.

•*DO NOT* try to remove an object you can't see, as you might push it farther into the ear canal.

•*DO NOT* try to wash an object out of the ear if there is the possibility that the object (such as dried beans or sponges) will absorb water and swell.

•*DO NOT* try to remove the object with tweezers if the victim is a young child. Leave it to medical personnel.

F–H

NOSE

•Try to get the victim to sneeze. Having the victim sniff black pepper or tickling his nose with a feather might help.

•If the object remains, ask the victim to blow gently into a tissue, while pinching shut the unaffected nostril.

•If you can see the object, try removing it with tweezers. *DO NOT* push it in farther.

•If you can't remove the object, seek medical care.

THROAT

•See Choking, page 67.

FRACTURES

See Broken Bones, page 50

FROSTBITE

Frostbite is the freezing of the skin and, in severe cases, the underlying tissue. It occurs when the body is exposed to below-freezing temperatures and most often affects the face, hands, ears, and feet.

Frostbite may be superficial, in which only the skin is frozen, or it can be deep, affecting the skin and the underlying tissue. No matter how severe the frostbite, the treatment is the same. By following the steps below in a careful manner, you can help prevent, or at least minimize, serious damage from frostbite, even if you're in a remote wilderness location.

What To Look For

SUPERFICIAL FROSTBITE

•Red, swollen skin that becomes white, waxy, or grayish yellow
•Affected area is cold and numb
•Stiff skin surface with soft tissue underneath
•Tingling or stinging when thawed

F–H

PREVENTION POINTERS

Fingers, toes, noses, and ears are all at risk for frostbite when the weather is cold. Always dress appropriately when enjoying the great outdoors. See pages 210 and 217.

DEEP FROSTBITE
- Affected area is cold, solid, and hard
- Loss of feeling in previously painful, cold area
- Blisters or swelling may appear when thawed
- Severe pain when thawed

What To Do (and Not To Do)
- Take the victim to a warm place. Remove any jewelry or clothing from the affected area.
- Give the victim warm drinks. *DO NOT* allow the victim to smoke or drink alcohol.
- Check for signs of dehydration and treat as necessary (see Dehydration, page 77).
- *DO NOT* massage the affected area or rub it with snow or cold water.
- If possible, call EMS or get the victim to a medical facility. If this isn't possible, you should rewarm the victim yourself (see Rewarming a Frostbite Victim, below).
- *DO NOT* attempt to warm the victim, until there is no risk of re-freezing. This is because most of the damage from frostbite occurs during the freezing and thawing process.
- After rewarming, cover the affected area with clean, dry dressings. Separate affected toes and fingers with dry, sterile gauze. *DO NOT* break any blisters that may appear.

F–H

REWARMING A FROSTBITE VICTIM

- Place the affected area in warm (102°F to 105°F), *not* hot, water. If you don't have a thermometer, check the temperature of the water on the inside of your lower arm. Keep adding warm water, to keep the temperature stable. *DO NOT* use direct heat, such as an open fire, hot water bottle or heater, to rewarm the victim.
- If the face or ears are frostbitten, soak clean cloths in warm water and place on the affected area. Replace the cloths often with newly warmed ones.
- Rewarming can be painful. Give the victim acetaminophen or ibuprofen or, if an adult, aspirin to ease the pain.
- Rewarming has been completed when the victim's tissue feels soft to the touch and sensation has returned.

•If possible, elevate the affected area above the victim's heart to reduce swelling.

•Get medical care for the frostbite victim as soon as possible.

GENITAL INJURY

The genital areas in both men and women are rich in nerve and blood supply. That's why injuries to this area can cause severe pain and bleeding.

Genital injuries are rarely life-threatening, but they are upsetting and painful for the victim. You can do much to treat and comfort the victim, as well as provide all-important privacy and, in cases of sexual assault, protect evidence. (See also Zipper Injuries, page 172.)

What To Look For
•Pain in the genital area
•Injury or wound in the genital area
•Bleeding
•Bruises and cuts
•Object embedded in a wound or body opening
•Rapid, weak pulse
•Pale, cold, clammy skin
•Sweating
•Weakness and dizziness
•Nausea and vomiting

What To Do (and Not To Do)

IF THE INJURY AND BLEEDING ARE NOT SEVERE

•Apply direct pressure to stop the bleeding and cover with a clean, dry dressing.

•Get medical help.

IF THE INJURY AND BLEEDING ARE SEVERE OR YOU THINK A SEXUAL ASSAULT HAS OCCURRED

•Check the victim's ABCs and treat as necessary (see page 9).

WHEN A CHILD SUFFERS GENITAL INJURY

There are other signs that may indicate a child has a genital injury. He may
•Refuse to go to the bathroom
•Rub or hold his genital area
•Complain of abdominal pain

CHECK

Airway
Breathing
Circulation

•Call 911 (EMS).

•Quickly provide comfort, support, and privacy for the victim.

•Ask unnecessary bystanders to leave.

•To help prevent shock, lay the victim down with legs elevated (this will increase blood flow to the heart and brain) and keep him warm with a blanket or coat (see page 147). *AVOID* moving the victim if a spinal cord injury is suspected (for more details, see page 154).

•Wash your hands with soap and water. Expose as little of the genital area as possible. *DO NOT* wash the wound and/or change the victim's clothing if a sexual assault is suspected; this is important to preserve evidence. *DO NOT* remove an embedded object if one is present; try to stabilize it by using dressings or bulky cloths.

•Place a sterile pad or clean cloth over the wound and apply direct, constant pressure. *DO NOT* apply direct pressure to an embedded object; press down firmly on either side of the injury. *DO NOT* remove blood-stained dressings; instead, place another on top to soak up the blood.

•If there is severe vaginal bleeding, you may need to pack the vagina with pads or clean cloths to stop the bleeding (see also page 169).

•Apply a covered ice pack or cold compress to the injured area, to reduce swelling.

•If any of the genitalia has been cut off, wrap it in moist, clean cloths. Sterile gauze is a good choice. Place the wrapped part in a clean plastic bag or wrap it in plastic wrap, and, if possible, put it into a container of slush (ice mixed with water). Be sure the ice never directly touches the amputated part. Label the container with the victim's name and time of the accident, and take it to the hospital with the victim.

F–H

HAND INJURIES

Like all parts of the body, hands and fingers can be exposed to a variety of injuries, such as cuts or cold exposure. But they are also particularly susceptible to other injuries, such as blood under the nail, damaged or torn-off nails, and crushed hands or fingers.

You can easily treat many hand and finger injuries at home, although others may require medical care.

See also Cuts (page 74), Puncture Wounds (page 133), Cold Exposure (page 73), and Frostbite (page 102).

What To Look For
- Partly or completely torn-off nail
- Blood under the nail
- Wound on finger or hand
- Pain and tenderness
- Swelling
- Bruising
- Twisted fingers
- Puncture site

What To Do (and Not To Do)

CRUSHED HAND OR FINGER
- Place an ice pack on the injured area to reduce swelling.
- Gently try to remove any rings from fingers. If rings are not easily removed, *DO NOT* force them.
- Control bleeding from the surface of hands or fingers by applying direct pressure with a clean cloth or gauze dressing (see Bleeding Under a Nail, page 107). Wash the wound with soap and water and cover with a clean, dry dressing. Keep the hand elevated above the level of the heart to prevent swelling or throbbing.
- Give the victim acetaminophen or ibuprofen or, if an adult, aspirin, to relieve pain.
- Check for pain, tenderness, and movement in the

bones and joints of the fingers. Seek immediate medical care if you suspect a broken bone (see page 50) or a dislocation (see page 83), or bleeding from the wound is severe or won't stop (see page 38).

•If a finger has been severed, call 911 (EMS) (see page 141).

BLEEDING UNDER A NAIL

•Place the injured finger in ice water or apply an ice pack; keep the victim's hand elevated.

•Apply a dressing to absorb blood and protect the victim's nail.

•Seek medical care. Medical personnel can relieve the pressure and pain by creating a hole in the surface of the nail.

DAMAGED OR TORN-OFF NAIL

•If the nail is damaged, hold it in place by wrapping it in gauze secured with adhesive tape.

•If the nail is partly or completely torn off, spread an antibiotic ointment on the area and cover with an adhesive bandage.

•Seek medical care.

HEAD INJURY

The scalp, skull, brain, blood vessels, and spine can be injured by blows to the head. Some head injuries are visible, such as cuts to the scalp, and can bleed profusely. Others, such as skull fractures or brain injuries, are not always easily detected.

All head injuries are potentially serious and may be associated with a spinal injury. When providing first aid for head injuries, always proceed carefully to protect the neck and spine.

What To Look For

SCALP INJURY

•Scalp wound
•Pain
•Bleeding
•Rapid, weak pulse

F-H

REPEATED HEAD INJURIES

Repeated minor head injuries may result in injury to the brain. Athletes, parents, and coaches should be aware of the latest recommendations on managing head injuries (see page 215).

•Pale, cold, clammy skin
•Sweating
•Skin around the mouth and lips is blue (see also page 15)
•Weakness and dizziness

FRACTURED SKULL
•Embedded object or penetrating wound
•Indentation in the skull
•Blood or pink, watery fluid (cerebrospinal fluid) leaking from ears or nose
•Discoloration around the eyes or behind the ears
•Pupils of unequal size
•Loss of consciousness

BRAIN INJURY
•Severe headache
•Problems with vision, such as seeing double
•Pupils of unequal size
•Blood or pink, watery fluid (cerebrospinal fluid) leaking from the ears or nose
•Weakness or paralysis
•Changes in behavior
•Severe vomiting
•Slowed breathing
•Seizures
•Loss of consciousness

What To Do (and Not To Do)

IF SCALP INJURY IS NOT SEVERE
•Wash your hands with soap and water.
•Control the bleeding by applying direct pressure.
•Wash the wound with soap and water.
•Cover with a clean, dry dressing.
•Seek medical care.

IF SCALP INJURY IS SEVERE OR SKULL FRACTURE OR BRAIN INJURY IS SUSPECTED
•Check the victim's ABCs and treat as necessary (see page 9).

F–H

CHECK

Airway

Breathing

Circulation

- Call 911 (EMS).
- Wash your hands with soap and water. *DO NOT* wash the wound.
- Place a sterile pad or clean cloth over the wound and apply direct, constant pressure. If a skull fracture or an embedded object is present, *DO NOT* apply direct pressure and *DO NOT* remove the embedded object; press down firmly on either side of the injury. *DO NOT* remove blood-stained dressings; instead, place another on top to soak up the blood.
- Apply a covered ice pack to the injured area, to reduce the swelling.
- With all head injuries, spinal cord damage may be possible. If you suspect a spinal cord injury, *NEVER* move the victim unless absolutely necessary. Keep the victim's neck still until EMS arrive by placing your hands on either side of the neck or by placing firm cushions there (see also Spinal Injury, page 154).
- Vomiting can happen at any time, so keep a container, such as a pail or pot, and a damp cloth nearby.
- If you don't suspect a spinal cord injury, turn the victim on his left side—this is called the recovery position (see page 11). It will help prevent further vomiting and allow fluids to drain from his mouth.

HEADACHE AND HEAD PAIN

Many sources of headache and head pain, including stress, heat, overexertion, eye strain, and allergies, are not cause for alarm and can be easily treated. In some cases, however, headache and head pain can be a symptom of something more serious, such as meningitis or brain injury.

How can you tell the difference? Severe, sudden, or persistent headache or head pain usually signals a more serious condition and should be checked by a doctor. But, when in doubt about the nature of the headache or head pain, always seek medical care.

F–H

What To Look For

•Location of the head pain
•Changes in pain when victim alters position
•Fever
•Nausea and vomiting
•Visual problems, including double vision
•Stiff neck
•Loss of balance
•Confusion
•Seizures
•Weakness on one side of the body

What To Do (and Not To Do)

•Have the victim lie down in a dark room.
•Give the victim fluids with acetaminophen or ibuprofen or, if an adult, aspirin.
•If the victim has a prescription autoinjector for migraines, help him use it.
•Vomiting can happen at any time, so keep a container, such as a pail or pot, and a damp cloth nearby.
•Seek medical attention if the above treatments do not help or the headache or head pain returns.

POSSIBLE HEAD INJURY

•Call 911 (EMS) or take the victim immediately to the emergency room—after you have checked and treated the victim's ABCs (see page 9)—if the headache or head pain is

•Sudden or severe

•Accompanied by fever, stiff neck, seizures, double vision, weakness on one side of the body, mental confusion, or loss of consciousness

•A new type of headache and the victim is more than 50 years old or is pregnant

•If the victim has a head injury, spinal cord damage may be possible (see also Head Injury, page 107, and Spinal Injury, page 154).
•If you do not suspect a spinal cord injury, have the victim lie in a comfortable position.

F-H

CHECK

AIRWAY

BREATHING

CIRCULATION

HEART ATTACK

A heart attack (myocardial infarction) occurs when there is a blockage (clot) in one of the arteries that supplies oxygen to the heart. Without this oxygen, the heart muscle may be damaged or even cease to beat (cardiac arrest).

It can be difficult to know if pain or pressure in the chest is due to a heart attack or another problem, such as indigestion or asthma. When in doubt, always seek emergency medical care. (See also Chest Pain, page 60)

Recognizing the signs of a heart attack and knowing how to give first aid properly, especially CPR (cardiopulmonary resuscitation, see page 12), can save lives.

What To Look For
•Pressure, squeezing, heaviness, or pain in the chest, usually behind the breastbone
•Pain that spreads to the shoulder, neck, lower jaw, down the arm, or into the back
•Shortness of breath
•Weak, rapid pulse
•Pale, cold, clammy skin
•Skin around the mouth and lips is blue (see also page 15)
•Weakness
•Nausea and vomiting
•Dizziness
•Anxiety
•Loss of consciousness

What To Do (and Not To Do)
•Call 911 (EMS) immediately. Determine whether an automated external defibrillator (see page 21) is available, in case you have to use it.
•Check the victim's ABCs and treat as necessary (see page 9).
•Give an aspirin to the victim to chew and swallow unless he has been told not to take aspirin.

FOR MORE INFORMATION...

The American Heart Association is a good source of information on preventing and treating heart disease. See page 250.

F–H

CHECK

Airway

Breathing

Circulation

•Place the heart attack victim in a comfortable, upright position.

•Calm and comfort the victim.

•If the victim normally takes a medication called nitroglycerin for chest pain, help him to place it under his tongue. The victim should be sitting or lying down to take this medication.

•If oxygen is available, such as in an airplane or dentist's office, give it to the victim.

•Continue to monitor the victim's ABCs every 10 minutes until EMS arrive.

PREVENTION POINTERS

Heat exhaustion can develop quickly if you're active in a hot environment. You can play it safe with a few sensible steps such as drinking plenty of fluids (in fact, more than you think you need) and resting if you feel overheated. See Sports Injuries, page 215.

HEAT EXHAUSTION

Sweating is a vital way for our bodies to stay cool. But when we sweat excessively and don't drink enough fluids, we can lose too much salt and water, resulting in heat exhaustion. This condition is usually caused by overexertion, particularly in hot weather, including working for long periods in hot, poorly ventilated offices.

In most cases, helping a victim of heat exhaustion is a simple exercise that will help the victim recover quickly and avoid developing the more serious condition of heatstroke (see page 113). See also Dehydration, page 77.

What To Look For
•Heavy sweating
•Severe thirst and dry tongue
•Pale, cold, clammy skin
•Cramps in the abdomen, legs, or arms
•Headache
•Rapid, weak pulse
•Nausea and vomiting
•Diarrhea
•Dizziness or faintness

What To Do (and Not To Do)
•Immediately move the victim to a cool place.

•Give the victim cool water or any other drink that is available. *AVOID* giving drinks containing caffeine or alcohol, and *DO NOT* give the victim salt tablets.

•Raise and support the victim's legs.

•Loosen any tight clothing.

•Fan the victim and place a cold compress on his forehead.

•If symptoms persist, seek medical care.

IF THE VICTIM LOSES CONSCIOUSNESS

•Check the victim's ABCs and treat as necessary (see page 9).

•Call 911 (EMS) and continue cooling the victim (see Heatstroke, below).

•Roll the victim onto his left side—this is called the recovery position (see page 11). It will help prevent vomiting and allow fluids to drain from his mouth.

CHECK

A IRWAY
B REATHING
C IRCULATION

F–H

HEATSTROKE

Heatstroke is a serious heat-related illness. In this condition, the sweat glands are unable to cool the body effectively (perhaps because of heat or an illness), and the body temperature rises to dangerously high levels.

Whenever heatstroke develops, it is an emergency situation that requires speedy first aid action.

What To Look For
•Body feels hot to the touch
•Flushed, dry skin
•Rapid pulse
•Headache
•Nausea, vomiting, diarrhea
•Changes in behavior such as confusion or aggression
•Staggering gait
•Seizures

DEHYDRATION AND HEATSTROKE

Dehydration (see page 77) and some medications can be a major contributor to the development of heatstroke, especially in the elderly. Athletes may be at risk of heatstroke if they can't sweat fast enough to cool their bodies (see Sports Injuries, page 215).

•Loss of consciousness

•Coma

What To Do (and Not To Do)

IF THE VICTIM IS CONSCIOUS

•Call 911 (EMS).

•Immediately remove as much of the victim's clothing as possible.

•Spray the victim with water, and fan him vigorously to promote cooling.

•If possible, immerse the victim in a shallow pool of cold water. *NEVER* leave the victim unattended in the water.

•Give him small amounts of cool liquids.

•Vomiting or diarrhea can happen at any time, so keep a container, such as a pail or pot, and a damp cloth nearby.

IF THE VICTIM IS UNCONSCIOUS OR LOSES CONSCIOUSNESS

•Check the victim's ABCs and treat as necessary (see page 9).

•Call 911 (EMS).

•Cool or continue to cool the victim (see above).

•Roll the victim onto his left side—this is called the recovery position (for details, see page 11). It will help prevent vomiting and allow fluids to drain from his mouth.

CHECK

Airway

Breathing

Circulation

HEIMLICH MANEUVER

See Choking, page 67

HIGH BLOOD PRESSURE

Blood pressure is the force needed to carry blood to all parts of the body. It is created by the force of the blood pushing against blood vessel walls. High blood pressure develops when this pressure becomes too great.

High blood pressure can be due to obesity, poor diet, or lack of regular exercise, or it can be hereditary. Stress and drinking large amounts of alcohol may play a role as well. Occasionally, high blood pressure is a sign of an illness or injury.

If left untreated, high blood pressure weakens blood vessel walls and damages organs, such as the heart. It is a leading cause of stroke (see page 159), heart attack (see page 111), and kidney failure. Measuring blood pressure on a regular basis is the only way to recognize high readings and, through treatment, prevent serious damage. If you or someone in hour household has high blood pressure, consider buying a home blood pressure kit so blood pressure can be monitored at home regularly.

What To Look For
•Onset without warning signs
•Headache
•Ringing in ears
•Dizziness
•Nosebleed
•Feeling of fullness in head
•Blood pressure reading of 140/90 to 160/95 (borderline high blood pressure)
•Blood pressure reading over 160/95 (high blood pressure)

What To Do (and Not To Do)
•Calm and reassure the victim. Repeat the blood pressure test after 15 minutes.
•Seek medical care if blood pressure exceeds 140/90.
•If medication is prescribed, have the victim take it as directed.
•Ensure the victim has regular checkups to monitor his blood pressure.

HOUSEHOLD POISONING
See Poisoning and Drug Overdose, page 131

LIFESTYLE CHANGES THAT HELP PREVENT OR CONTROL HIGH BLOOD PRESSURE

•Losing weight, if overweight
•Exercising regularly
•Drinking alcohol in moderation
•Stopping smoking
•Eating a healthy diet and limiting salt intake

F–H

HYPERVENTILATION

Hyperventilation—deep, fast breathing—occurs when a victim is feeling out of breath and increases the rate at which he breathes. As this rapid breathing continues, the victim gets rid of too much carbon dioxide, causing muscle tightness in the chest and throat, as well as tingling, numbness, and cramping in the hands and feet.

Hyperventilation is often caused by stress and anxiety, although it can result from conditions such as asthma, uncontrolled diabetes, or head injury. You can treat and reverse hyperventilation with a few simple steps.

What To Look For
•Rapid, deep breathing
•Shortness of breath
•Dizziness or faintness
•Tingling, numbness, or cramping of the hands and feet
•Numbness around the mouth
•Anxiety

What To Do (and Not To Do)
•Calm the victim.
•Encourage the victim to slow his breathing. Using his abdominal muscles, the victim should inhale through the nose, hold his breath for a few seconds, and then slowly exhale through pursed lips.
•If that doesn't work, the victim can try breathing in and out of a paper (not plastic) bag for a short time, while you reassure him.
•If the symptoms continue, seek medical attention.
•If you suspect that the hyperventilation may be due to an injury or illness, seek immediate medical attention.

F–H

HYPOTHERMIA

Hypothermia is a condition that develops when the body loses more heat than it produces and the core temperature drops below 95°F. Hypothermia often results from exposure to below-freezing temperatures and may be accompanied by frostbite (see page 102). However, this condition can also develop in warmer temperatures, under such conditions as wind or wet clothing, or if the victim is inactive.

Hypothermia can be a life-threatening situation but can often be reversed if action is taken in its early stages.

What To Look For

MILD HYPOTHERMIA
• Body temperature is between 91°F and 95°F.
• Shivering
• Cold, pale skin
• Strange behavior, such as confusion or aggressiveness
• Cool abdomen
• Cramps
• Stiff muscles

SEVERE HYPOTHERMIA
• Body temperature below 90°F
• Shivering stops
• Unresponsive
• Slow, weak pulse
• Fixed pupils (pupils that do not respond to light)
• Loss of consciousness
• Heart stops beating

What To Do (and Not To Do)
• Take the victim to a warm place. Be sure to handle the victim carefully. Rough handling can cause the heart to stop beating.

DEHYDRATION

Be aware that exposure to cold temperatures often leads to dehydration (see page 77).

F–H

•Remove all wet clothes and replace with warm, dry clothes.
•Lay the victim flat. *DO NOT* elevate his legs.

IF THE VICTIM HAS MILD HYPOTHERMIA
•You may begin warming the victim by using blankets, heaters, and/or covered hot water bottles, or by sharing your own body heat. *DO NOT* massage the victim's body.
•Give the victim a warm drink containing sugar. *AVOID* giving drinks containing caffeine or alcohol.

IF HYPOTHERMIA IS SEVERE
•Check the victim's ABCs and treat as necessary (see page 9). Be aware that the breathing and pulse in a victim with hypothermia may be faint and hard to detect. That's why it's important to take 30 to 45 seconds to check the victim's breathing and pulse before starting CPR.
•Call 911 (EMS) immediately and begin warming the victim as above.

CHECK

Airway

Breathing

Circulation

I–M

PREVENTION POINTERS

Using insect repellent and wearing proper attire is the best way to avoid being stung by an insect. For more details, see Hiking and Camping, page 209.

INSECT STINGS

Insects, including bees, wasps, hornets, and fire ants, inject venom using their stingers. Unlike wasps and hornets, bees leave their stingers behind, and they may continue to release venom into a victim's body.

Insects stings can be painful and sometimes scary, but usually they cause only a mild reaction that is relieved by simple measures. However, if a person has been stung in the mouth or throat, or if he is allergic to the venom, a more serious allergic reaction can occur. If left untreated, a severe allergic reaction can lead to anaphylactic shock, a life-threatening condition that causes swelling of the airway and stops the victim's ability to breathe.

Be on the lookout for signs of a serious allergic reaction and anaphylactic shock. By acting promptly and obtaining immediate medical attention, you can help save a victim's life.

What To Look For

MILD REACTION
•Warmth, burning pain, swelling, or redness at the sting site.
•Flushing in the face, neck, hands, feet, or tongue
•Hives (blotchy, raised rash)

SEVERE ALLERGIC REACTION
Any of the above signs plus the following:
•Tightness in chest or throat
•Rapid breathing
•Skin around the mouth and lips is blue (see also page 15)
•Nausea and/or vomiting
•Abdominal pain
•Pale, damp skin
•Anxiety

ANAPHYLACTIC SHOCK
Any of the above signs plus the following:
•Wheezing or difficulty breathing
•Feeling faint, drowsiness
•Loss of consciousness

What To Do (and Not To Do)

MILD REACTION
•If the victim was stung by a bee, search for the stinger in the skin and remove it. Scrape the stinger away with your fingernail, knife blade, or credit card. *DO NOT* use tweezers. A stinger may release more poison if it is squeezed by tweezers.
•Using soap and water, wash the sting site and cover it with a cold compress or ice pack. If possible, keep the sting site below the level of the victim's heart.
•To reduce the stinging pain, apply a paste of baking soda and water.
•To relieve itching and swelling, apply calamine lotion. Consider giving the victim Benadryl

I–M

(diphenhydramine hydrochloride) if he can swallow and has taken Benadryl before.

•Monitor the victim for an allergic reaction. A delayed reaction can develop up to 24 hours after the victim has been stung by a bee.

•Keep an eye on the sting site for 2 to 3 days. If it becomes infected (redness, swelling, tenderness, or fever), take the victim to the doctor.

SEVERE ALLERGIC REACTION AND ANAPHYLACTIC SHOCK

•Check the victim's ABCs and treat as necessary (see page 9).

•If an epinephrine kit is available, inject epinephrine according to instructions. More than one dose may be needed to reverse the anaphylactic shock.

•Call 911 (EMS). Look for a card or medical identification bracelet that contains information about the victim's allergies.

•If the insect-sting victim uses an asthma inhaler, help him use it.

•Consider giving the victim Benadryl (diphenhydramine hydrochloride) if he can swallow and has taken Benadryl before.

•To help prevent shock, lay the victim down with legs elevated (this will increase blood flow to the heart and brain) and keep him warm with a blanket or coat (see page 147).

•If the victim is having trouble breathing, place him in a sitting position.

•If the victim was stung by a bee, search for the stinger in the skin and remove it (as above).

•Comfort the victim and help him stay calm while you're waiting for EMS.

•*AVOID* giving the victim food or drink.

INTERNAL BLEEDING

See Bleeding-Internal, page 41

CHECK

Airway

Breathing

Circulation

I–M

LYME DISEASE
See Tick Bites, page 166

MARINE ANIMAL BITES AND STINGS

Many types of animals living in our waters can bite or sting. Sharks, barracudas, jellyfish, Portuguese man-of-wars, coral, anemones, stingrays, and cone shells are just some of the marine animals that can deliver poisonous venom to the body.

Most bites and stings are easily treated, although you should keep an eye out for a severe allergic reaction.

What To Look For

MILD ALLERGIC REACTION
•Warmth, burning pain, swelling, or redness at the sting site
•Retained parts from the marine animal (such as jellyfish tentacles) at the contact site
•Flushing in the face, neck, hands, feet, or tongue
•Hives (blotchy, raised rash)

SEVERE ALLERGIC REACTION
Any of the above signs plus the following:
•Tightness in chest or throat
•Rapid breathing
•Skin around the mouth and lips is blue (see also page 15)
•Nausea and/or vomiting
•Abdominal pain
•Pale, damp skin
•Anxiety

ANAPHYLACTIC SHOCK
Any of the above signs plus the following:
•Wheezing or difficulty breathing

I–M

•Feeling faint, drowsiness
•Loss of consciousness

What To Do (and Not To Do)

(SEE ALSO TREATMENT FOR SPECIFIC BITES AND STINGS, PAGE 123)

•Remove any jewelry or clothing covering the injured area.
•Keep the victim still, and place the injured area below the level of his heart to help prevent the venom from spreading throughout the body.
•If there is bleeding, take steps to control it. Always wash your hands before and after caring for the victim.

IF THE BLEEDING IS NOT SEVERE
•Apply direct pressure to stop the bleeding.
•Wash the wound with soap and water.
•Cover with a clean, dry dressing.

IF THE BLEEDING IS SEVERE
•Check the victim's ABCs and treat as necessary (see page 9).
•Call 911 (EMS).
•Place a sterile pad or clean cloth over the wound and apply direct, constant pressure.
•If an embedded object or a protruding bone is present, *DO NOT* apply direct pressure. Press down firmly on either side of the injury.
•If the bleeding doesn't stop, apply harder pressure with both hands over a greater area. *DO NOT* remove blood-stained dressings; instead, place another dressing on top to soak up the blood.
•If the bleeding continues, apply pressure at the victim's pressure points (see page 40).

SEVERE ALLERGIC REACTION AND ANAPHYLACTIC SHOCK

•Check the victim's ABCs and treat as necessary (see page 9).

CHECK

Airway
Breathing
Circulation

I-M

TREATMENT FOR SPECIFIC BITES AND STINGS

STINGS (PORTUGUESE MAN-OF-WARS, JELLYFISH, CORALS, ANEMONES)

•Rinse the site with salt water, and apply vinegar.

•Scrape the area with a plastic card, comb, or knife blade (this prevents remnants of the tentacles from injecting more poison). Tweezers can be used to remove large tentacles. *DO NOT* remove tentacles with your bare hands.

•Soak the sting site in vinegar for 15 to 30 minutes (until pain goes away).

•Note: Meat tenderizer has not been shown to be beneficial for these injuries.

PUNCTURES (STING RAYS, CONE SHELLS)

•Rinse the wound with salt water to remove any venom.

•Control bleeding by applying direct pressure (see page 122).

•Soak the puncture wound in hot water for 30 to 90 minutes. The water should be as hot as possible (110°F to 113°F) without burning the victim.

•Apply a clean, dry dressing.

•Seek medical care.

BITES (SHARKS, BARRACUDAS, EELS)

•Check the victim's ABCs and treat as necessary (see page 9).

•Control bleeding by applying direct pressure (see page 122).

•Seek immediate medical care as required.

•If an epinephrine kit is available, inject epinephrine according to instructions. More than one dose may be needed to reverse the anaphylactic shock.

•Call 911 (EMS). Look for a card or medical identification bracelet that contains information about the victim's allergies.

•To help prevent shock, lay the victim down with legs elevated (this will increase blood flow to the heart and brain) and keep him warm with a blanket or coat (see page 147). If the victim is having trouble breathing, place him in a sitting position. *AVOID* moving the victim if a spinal cord injury is suspected (see page 154).

•*AVOID* giving the victim food or drink.

•Consider giving the victim Benadryl (diphenhydramine hydrochloride) if he can swallow and has taken Benadryl before.

•Comfort the victim and help him stay calm while you're waiting for EMS.

M–I

MISCARRIAGE

See Vaginal Bleeding, page 169

MOUNTAIN SICKNESS

See Altitude Sickness, page 33

MUSCLE INJURY

Strains, bruising, and cramps are the most common types of muscle injury (see also page 157). A muscle strain is caused by an awkward unexpected movement or by a severe jarring motion during a sports activity. Muscle bruising (contusion) usually results from a direct blow. Muscle cramps, on the other hand, are the result of an internal process, such as a body chemical imbalance, or when the body lacks water to get rid of waste products.

Muscles throughout the body, such as those in the legs, arms, stomach, shoulder, neck, and back, are at risk of injury. Appropriate first aid, including the use of RICE (rest, ice, compression, and elevation; see page 158) can help speed recovery time and return the victim to his regular activities.

What To Look For

MUSCLE STRAINS
• Pain, tenderness, and stiffness at the site of injury
• Indentation or bump
• Weakness and loss of function

MUSCLE BRUISES (CONTUSIONS)
• Pain and tenderness in injured area
• Black and blue marks

MUSCLE SPASMS
•Severe pain
•Reduced or no movement at site of spasm

What To Do (and Not To Do)

MUSCLE STRAINS AND BRUISES
•Start the RICE procedure right away (see page 158)
•Apply heat after 48 to 72 hours.
•Give the victim ibuprofen or, if an adult, aspirin, to relieve the pain and inflammation of the muscle injury.
•If injury is severe or doesn't improve, seek medical assistance.

MUSCLE CRAMPS
•Ask the victim to stop what he's doing.
•Gently stretch the victim's affected muscle.
•Apply pressure and ice to relax the muscle. *DO NOT* rub or massage the muscle, because you might increase the pain.
•Give the victim a commercial sports drink that contains a balanced electrolyte solution (such as Gatorade).
•If the cramps persist, seek medical assistance.

NOSE INJURY

The nose is a sensitive area, with many nerves and blood vessels. That's why injuries to the nose can be painful, bloody, and upsetting for the victim. What's more, they can interfere with breathing.

Blood or fluid flowing from the nose may indicate a severe head injury. But, in general, bleeding from the nose is a common feature of nose injuries and not a sign of anything serious.

What To Look For
•Pain and swelling
•Bleeding from the nose or cuts on the nose

N–R

•Eye area is bruised

•Nose appears crooked or bent out of shape

What To Do (and Not To Do)

•If you suspect a head or neck injury, call 911 (EMS).

•Have the victim sit down.

•If there is bleeding from the nose, ask the victim to lean forward. Apply firm direct pressure (see Nosebleed, below).

•If there is bleeding from a cut on the nose, control it by applying direct pressure and cover with a clean, dry dressing.

•Check if a foreign object has become stuck in the nose. If so, remove it (see page 99).

•Apply a cold compress or covered ice pack to the nose.

•Seek medical care.

NOSEBLEED

A nosebleed is usually caused by a broken blood vessel in the septum (the structure that divides the nostrils). Colds, nose picking, dry air, allergies, or a blow to the nose are just a few of the reasons a nosebleed occurs.

A serious, less common form of nosebleed involves bleeding into the back of the mouth and throat. This type of nosebleed requires immediate medical attention.

Most nosebleeds involve bleeding in the front of the nose, with the blood flowing out of the nose through one nostril. These types of nosebleeds are usually not serious and can often be treated successfully at home.

What To Look For

•Bleeding from the nose or into the back of the mouth and throat

---

PREVENTION POINTERS

Using a room humidifier can prevent nosebleeds that are caused by heated, dry air.

N–R

•Gagging, choking, coughing, nausea, or vomiting due to bleeding into the throat

•Signs of bleeding from other sites, such as the gums, in the absence of a traumatic injury

What To Do (and Not To Do)

•Ask the victim to sit up and lean slightly forward.

•Encourage the victim to breathe through his mouth.

•Using a tissue or gauze, firmly pinch the lower, fleshy end of the nose together for 5 minutes. Maintain even pressure.

•Get medical help if the above steps don't stop the bleeding, if the bleeding is into the back of the mouth and throat, or if you suspect a broken nose.

•Seek immediate medical care if there is bleeding from other sites, such as the gums, in the absence of traumatic injury—this indicates a dangerous medical problem.

IF YOU SUSPECT A SEVERE HEAD OR NECK INJURY OR THE VICTIM IS UNCONSCIOUS

•Check the victim's ABCs and treat as necessary (see page 9).

•Call 911 (EMS).

•With all head and neck injuries, spinal cord damage may be possible. *NEVER* move the victim, if you suspect a spinal cord injury, unless absolutely necessary. Keep the victim's neck still until the arrival of EMS by placing your hands on either side of the neck or by placing firm cushions there. (See also Head Injury, page 107, and Spinal Injury, page 154.)

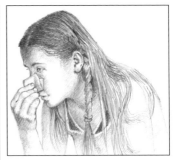

Pinching the nose to stop it from bleeding.

CHECK

Airway

Breathing

Circulation

N–R

OBJECTS IN THE EYES, EARS, NOSE, OR THROAT

See Foreign Objects in the Eye, Ear, Nose, or Throat, page 99

PELVIC PAIN

The pelvis is a cavity in the lower abdomen enclosed by a bony ring. It contains the lower part of the gastrointestinal tract, female reproductive organs, and bladder.

Pain in the pelvis can be caused by many different conditions—menstruation in women of reproductive age, uterine bleeding in postmenopausal women, and ovarian tumors. Other conditions, such as bladder problems or sexually transmitted diseases, can cause pelvic pain in both men and women.

Pelvic pain can also signal an injury caused by a blow or fall. Pelvic injuries, particularly fractures, are serious and require emergency treatment.

What To Look For
•Tenderness and pain in the pelvis, hips, back, or groin (where the lower abdomen meets the inner part of the thigh)
•Feeling of having to urinate
•Swollen or rigid abdomen
•Nausea and vomiting
•Diarrhea
•Fever
•Signs of internal bleeding—black, tarry stools, vomiting of blood, or bruising on the abdomen
•Loss of function in legs

What To Do (and Not To Do)
•Have the victim lie down in a comfortable position with knees bent.
•Heat applied to the abdomen can help relieve the pain. Place a covered hot water bottle on the victim's abdomen.
•Vomiting can happen at any time, so keep a container, such as a pail or pot, and a damp cloth nearby.
•Give the victim acetaminophen or ibuprofen or, if an adult, aspirin, to relieve pain. *AVOID* giving the victim food or drink until you have consulted a doctor.

•If pain is severe or persists, seek medical care.

•If the victim is or may be pregnant, seek immediate medical care. Pelvic pain may be a sign of a ruptured fallopian tube caused by an ectopic pregnancy (pregnancy that develops outside the uterus).

IF YOU SUSPECT A PELVIC INJURY

•Check the victim's ABCs and treat as necessary (see page 9).

•Call 911 (EMS).

•Lay the victim down on a firm surface.

•Immobilize the injured pelvis by placing pads between the victim's thighs and tying the legs together at knees and ankles.

•To help prevent shock, lay the victim down with legs elevated (this will increase blood flow to the heart and brain) and keep him warm with a blanket or coat (see page 147). *AVOID* moving the victim if a spinal cord injury is suspected (for more details, see page 154).

•If the victim vomits, carefully log-roll him onto his left side (see page 155). Support his head and neck and roll the body as one unit. If possible, have three or more people help you do this.

> **CHECK**
>
> **A**IRWAY
> **B**REATHING
> **C**IRCULATION

POISON IVY, OAK, AND SUMAC

Poison ivy, oak, and sumac are related plants, found throughout the United States, that can cause an allergic reaction when a person comes into contact with their oil or resin. The reaction can be mild or severe depending on the sensitivity of the victim.

A rash usually develops within 24 to 48 hours and may last for a few days or even a few weeks. This rash isn't contagious and can't be spread once the oil has been washed off.

Simple first aid measures will usually treat the rash and relieve the itching. Your best defense against poison ivy, oak, and sumac is recognizing and avoiding these plants, as well as wearing long

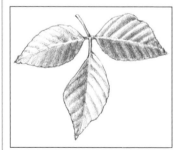

Poison ivy

N–R

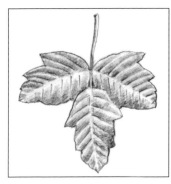

Poison oak

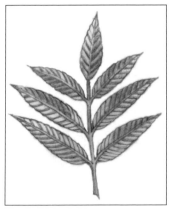

Poison sumac

N–R

pants and sleeves to prevent immediate contact with the skin. There are preventive lotions available, which provide a barrier against the toxic resin from plants and may prevent skin infection from occurring. Applied like a sunscreen to all exposed skin before going outside, this lotion guards against the harmful oil in poison ivy, oak, and sumac.

What To Look For

- Itching
- Redness
- Rash
- Blisters
- Swelling
- Possible infection, with tenderness and pus in the exposed area

What To Do (and Not To Do)

- As soon as you know the victim has been exposed to the plant, immediately wash the area with soap and water. Run the water for several minutes, so the plant oil is completely removed. Clean under the victim's fingernails as well. *DO NOT* spread the plant oil by rubbing or wiping the affected area.
- Wash the victim's clothing as well as anything else (such as a backpack and shoes and shoelaces) that may have come into contact with the plant. Remember that clothing and other items that have plant residue on them can cause a reaction months or years later.
- To relieve the itching in the victim's affected area, you might
    - Apply a drying lotion (such as calamine lotion)
    - Consider giving an antihistamine, such as Benadryl (diphenhydramine hydrochloride), if the victim has taken it before
    - Have the victim take a tepid bath containing 2 cups of colloid oatmeal (which is available in any drugstore)
- *DO NOT* let the victim scratch the rash.

•If the rash is severe or persists, or an infection develops, seek medical care.

POISONING AND DRUG OVERDOSE

A poison is a substance that damages the body, either temporarily or permanently. Poisons can enter the body in a variety of ways—by breathing, swallowing, or injection or absorption through the person's skin.

Many household chemicals and medications may be dangerous if accidentally ingested, or, if a medication, taken in more than the recommended dose.

Poisoning can also be caused by intentional drug abuse and overdose both at home and away from home. People under the influence of drugs can be difficult or even dangerous, but they are still in need of help. Knowing how to provide this help in an effective and safe manner (both for you and the victim) is key.

When a poisoning occurs, either intentionally or accidentally, quick but considered action will help prevent or lessen damage to the victim.

What To Look For

HOUSEHOLD CHEMICAL POISONING
•Open containers of chemical poison
•Burns or blisters on the lips and mouth
•Burns on other body parts where the chemical may have spilled
•Unexplained stains on skin or clothing
•Chest pain, difficulty breathing
•Nausea and vomiting
•Headache
•Large or small pupils
•Pale, cold, clammy skin
•Abdominal pain or cramps
•Diarrhea
•Weakness and confusion

PREVENTION POINTERS

There are many ways you can protect your family from poisonings. Keeping a close eye on your children is an important step. So, too, is properly storing and using all household chemicals and medications in your home (see Preventing Poisonings, page 186).

N–R

•Drowsiness

•Seizures

•Loss of consciousness

DRUG OVERDOSE

•Empty bottles or containers on or near the person

•Needle marks on skin

•Large or small pupils

•Drowsiness

•Anxiety, confusion, wild behavior

•Sweating

•Hallucinations

•Nausea and vomiting

•Headache

•Weak, irregular pulse or rapid pulse

•Seizures

•Loss of consciousness

•Coma

What To Do (and Not To Do)

•Check the victim's ABCs and treat as necessary (see page 9).

•Call 911 (EMS) if the victim is having trouble breathing, is having seizures, or is unconscious. Otherwise, call a poison control center.

•If the victim has swallowed a corrosive chemical, give 1 to 2 glasses of water or milk, if the victim is conscious. *DO NOT* give vinegar or baking soda in an attempt to neutralize the chemical.

•Give EMS or the poison control center as much information as you can about what's happened:

•The type or name of poison or medication

•When it was taken and how much

•Details on the victim: age, weight, and current condition

•Follow the instructions of the poison control center or EMS. *DO NOT* rely on the instructions found on the container's label.

•*DO NOT* make the victim vomit unless you are advised to do so by either the poison control center or EMS.

CHECK

Airway

Breathing

Circulation

N–R

•Assess the victim for any injuries and treat as required.

•To help prevent shock, lay the victim down with legs elevated (this will increase blood flow to the heart and brain) and keep him warm with a blanket or coat (see page 147). *AVOID* moving the victim if a spinal cord injury is suspected (see page 154).

•If the victim is vomiting or drooling, turn him onto his left side. This is called the recovery position (see page 11) and will help prevent further vomiting and allow fluids to drain from his mouth. If you suspect a spinal cord injury, carefully log-roll him onto his left side, supporting his head and neck and keeping his head in line with his body. If possible, have three or more people help you do this (see page 155).

•If the victim has been out in the cold for some time, hypothermia (see page 117) may be possible. Move the victim to a warmer place (unless he isn't breathing or may have a spinal injury), remove any wet clothing, and wrap him in warm blankets.

FOR VICTIMS OF DRUG OVERDOSE

•*DO NOT* stay with the victim if he becomes violent. You must consider your own safety as well. Move to a safer place and call the police.

•Try to determine whether the victim has also taken alcohol. Look for empty bottles on or near the person. Mixing drugs and alcohol is highly dangerous. If you suspect that this has occurred, be sure to tell EMS or the poison control center.

•Be aware that the victim may experience withdrawal after drug use has stopped. Signs of withdrawal from drugs are agitation, abdominal pain, confusion, hallucinations, shaking, and a strong desire for more of the drug. If you notice these signs, seek medical care for the victim.

PUNCTURE WOUNDS

Puncture wounds are small, deep holes made by a nail, knife, pin, or other object that can penetrate the

N–R

FISHHOOK INJURY

Fishhook injuries are a common occurrence and everyone who goes fishing should be prepared to remove a hook. Keep a pair of pliers and wire cutters in your tacklebox.

•*DO NOT* try to remove an embedded fishhook that is near the eye or near an artery.

•For superficial injuries in which only the point of the hook has entered the skin (not the barb), simply back the hook out of the skin and wash the wound.

•For injuries in which the barb is embedded in the skin, cut the eye of the hook, where the line is tied to the hook, with a pair of pliers or wire cutters; then advance the hook until the tip emerges from the skin. Grab the hook with your pliers and pull the hook out. Wash the wound and seek medical care as needed.

•Make sure the victim's tetanus immunization is up to date.

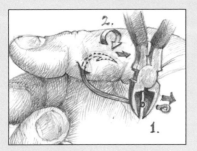

Cutting the eye of the hook when the barb is embedded in the skin.

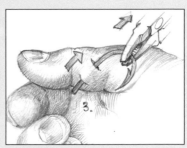

Advancing the hook and then removing with pliers.

DIABETES AND PUNCTURE WOUNDS

If the victim has diabetes or any blood disorders, consult a doctor about the puncture wound, because these victims are at higher risk of infection.

skin. Normally, punctures don't cause severe external bleeding wounds, although they can damage the skin and organs underneath. (See also Cuts, page 74.) However, if the object causing the puncture wound hits an artery, vein, or muscle, it can cause internal damage and bleeding (see page 41).

The risk of infection is high for puncture wounds, particularly if the wound was caused by a dirty object. That's why it's important to not only treat the wound, but also to find out whether the victim's tetanus immunization is up to date.

What To Look For

•Bleeding from an open wound
•Embedded object in the wound
•Redness, warmth, and swelling. These are signs of

infection, which can occur 24 to 48 hours after the injury. Be aware that swelling may also be a sign of internal injury (see below).

INTERNAL INJURY (DEEP PUNCTURE WOUND)
- Swelling
- Pain
- Blue discoloration to the skin
- Shock can develop (see page 146)

What To Do (and Not To Do)
- Wash your hands with soap and water.
- Locate the site of the bleeding. If necessary, remove or cut the victim's clothing.

IF THE PUNCTURE WOUND IS MINOR
- With tweezers, remove embedded objects that are in the top layer of skin.
- Apply direct pressure to stop the bleeding.
- Wash the wound with soap and water.
- Cover with a clean, dry dressing.
- Watch for signs of infection (pain, tenderness, pus, and red streaks). Seek medical care if necessary.
- Check the victim's tetanus immunization status. If it's not up to date, the victim may need to get a tetanus shot.

IF THE PUNCTURE WOUND IS DEEP AND SEVERE
- Check the victim's ABCs and treat as necessary (see page 9).
- Call 911 (EMS).
- Wash the wound with soap and water. *DO NOT* remove an object that is embedded in a wound. Secure it in place with bulky dressings.
- If there is bleeding from the wound, take steps to control it (see External Bleeding, page 38), including applying direct pressure, elevating the wound above the victim's heart level, pressing on the victim's pressure points, and applying a pressure bandage.

N–R

CHECK

AIRWAY

BREATHING

CIRCULATION

•To apply a pressure bandage, wrap a roller gauze bandage or long cloth tightly over the dressing, both above and below the wound. Split the bandage end into two strips; then knot the ends tightly, directly over the wound.
•A pressure bandage should be tight enough to keep pressure on the wound, but not so tight that it cuts off circulation. A bandage is too tight if there is no pulse beyond the wound (away from the victim's trunk), or if the skin in that area is turning blue.
•Check the victim's tetanus immunization status. If it's not up to date, the victim may need to get a tetanus shot.

FOR MORE INFORMATION...

Although cases of rabies in humans is rare in the United States, rabies continues to be a major health problem in many parts of the world. The Centers for Disease Control and Prevention Web site (page 257) is a good source of information on rabies, including facts on what precautions need to be taken before traveling to different areas.

RABIES

Rabies is the most dangerous viral infection caused by a bite from an animal. While the disease is rare in humans in the United States, it still exists in nonimmunized stray dogs and cats and in wild animals, including skunks, raccoons, and bats. In the United States, most cases of the disease in humans are from bat bites, and people may be unaware that they have been bitten by a bat. Rodents, such as mice and rats, do not carry or transmit rabies.

Rabies is transferred through an infected animal's saliva when it bites or licks the open wound on another animal or human. The rabies virus invades the nervous system and, eventually, the brain. This process takes 10 days to many months after the initial bite. Treatment is available for rabies but, to work, it must begin *before* symptoms appear. That's why you must take immediate action if you suspect that someone has been bitten by an animal that could be rabid, including any dog or cat with unknown immunization status.

What To Look For

A rabid animal may exhibit the following signs:
•Unprovoked attack
•Strange behavior—unusually aggressive or withdrawn

- Muscle spasms
- Inability to drink
- Extreme aversion to fluids
- Vomiting
- Paralysis

What To Do (and Not To Do)

IF THE VICTIM HAS BEEN BITTEN BY A HEALTHY DOMESTIC DOG OR CAT

- Provide first aid for the victim's bite (see Cat, Dog, and Other Animal Bites, page 56).
- Contact the owners to determine the animal's rabies immunization status. If the animal is immunized, there is no concern for rabies. If the animal is not immunized or its owners are unknown, it will have to be quarantined and watched for 10 days, to determine whether rabies is present.
- Report the biting incident to the police.

IF THE VICTIM HAS BEEN BITTEN BY A WILD OR STRAY ANIMAL OR BY ANY ANIMAL THAT HAS OR IS SUSPECTED TO HAVE RABIES

- Assume the animal has rabies. Seek immediate medical treatment. The victim will require a series of 5 rabies vaccine injections. To be effective, these injections must begin before symptoms appear in the victim.
- *DO NOT* attempt to capture the animal. Notify the police or animal control to capture and kill the animal.

SCORPION STINGS

Several types of scorpion live in the United States, primarily in the Southwest. This lobster-like creature (though much smaller) has a painful sting, but it generally isn't dangerous. The bark scorpion is one exception. Its sting is harmful to humans, especially children, and can cause a severe reaction that requires immediate medical care.

By keeping close watch on the victim and responding when a severe reaction develops, you

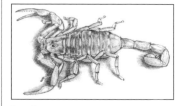

Scorpion

can help prevent a serious sting from taking a fatal course.

What To Look For

MILD REACTION
•Instant pain and burning at the sting site
•Numbness or tingling

SEVERE REACTION
•Severe pain
•Paralysis
•Uncontrolled twitching
•Rapid pulse
•Increased salivation
•Difficulty breathing
•Seizures
•Heart stops beating

What To Do (and Not To Do)
•Check the victim's ABCs and treat as necessary (see page 9).
•Carefully wash the sting site with soap and water.
•Apply a covered ice pack or cold compress, to reduce swelling at the sting site.
•Seek medical care.

IF THE REACTION IS OR BECOMES SEVERE
•Call 911 (EMS) and continue to monitor the ABCs until EMS arrive.
•To help prevent shock, lay the victim down with legs elevated (this will increase blood flow to the heart and brain) and keep him warm with a blanket or coat (see page 147). *AVOID* moving the victim if a spinal cord injury is suspected (for more details, see page 154).
•If the victim is having trouble breathing, place him in a sitting position.
•Comfort the victim and help him stay calm while you're waiting for EMS.
•*DO NOT* give the victim food or drink.

CHECK

Airway

Breathing

Circulation

S

SEIZURE

A seizure (convulsion) occurs when brain cells are stimulated in an abnormal way. The associated signs and symptoms depend on which part of the brain is stimulated.

Abnormal stimulation of the brain is caused by an underlying condition or injury, such as stroke, high fever in children, eclampsia (a complication of pregnancy), head injury, or poisoning. Epilepsy is a condition of repeated seizures, the cause of which may not be known.

In some cases, severe seizures, or those of an unknown origin, will require immediate medical care. Fortunately, most seizures do not need medical treatment. Your main role is to help prevent injury during the event and to comfort the victim when it's over.

What To Look For

NONMOTOR SEIZURE OR BEFORE A MOTOR SEIZURE
• Hearing strange sounds
• Taste sensations such as metallic taste in mouth
• Hallucinations
• Sense of déjà vu
• Confusion or altered mental status

NOT ALL SEIZURES ARE THE SAME

Seizures, like many medical conditions, can range in severity and symptoms.

NONMOTOR SEIZURE
On the milder end of the scale is a seizure that involves an altered mental status (such as brief lapse of attention) but no body twitching. This is called a nonmotor (for example, *petit mal*) seizure and usually lasts only a few seconds.

MOTOR SEIZURE
When a victim experiences jerky movements of the body, which may be associated with drooling or breathing difficulties, he is having a motor seizure. A motor seizure can involve one limb (focal seizure) or the entire body (grand mal seizure). Often there will be warning signs that a motor seizure is on its way.

S

MOTOR SEIZURE
- Body stiffness
- Jerky movement of face and limbs
- Eyes roll upward
- Drooling
- Loss of bladder or bowel control
- Breathing difficulties
- Loss of consciousness

AFTER A SEIZURE
- Confusion
- Memory loss
- Sleepiness

What To Do (and Not To Do)

NONMOTOR SEIZURE
- If you suspect the victim is having a nonmotor seizure, seek medical attention.

MOTOR SEIZURE
- If the victim senses that a seizure is approaching, have him sit or lie down to prevent a fall.
- If the victim is not already lying down, place him on the floor. Ask unnecessary bystanders to leave.
- Check whether the victim is wearing a medical alert bracelet or necklace.
- Loosen any tight clothing, especially around the victim's neck.
- If you *do not* suspect a spinal injury, place the victim on his left side—this is called the recovery position and will allow fluids to drain from his mouth (see page 11).
- If you do suspect a spinal injury, carefully log-roll him onto his left side. Support his head and neck, keep his head in line with his body, and roll the body as one unit. If possible, have three or more people help you do this (see page 155).
- Try to protect the victim from injuring himself during the seizure, but *DO NOT* hold him down.

•*DO NOT* place anything between the victim's teeth. (He will not swallow his tongue!)

•*DO NOT* give the victim anything to eat or drink. But if the victim has diabetes, put a sugar cube under his tongue.

AFTER A MOTOR SEIZURE

•Most seizures will be over in a few minutes, but be prepared for a second seizure to occur.

•Check the victim for any injuries that may have occurred during the seizure, and treat as required.

•In most cases, the victim will not need medical attention following a seizure.

•Allow the victim to sleep.

CALL 911 (EMS) IF

•The victim does not have epilepsy. It's important for medical personnel to determine what has caused the seizure.

•The victim has a second seizure directly after the first one.

•The victim appears ill or is injured.

•The victim is pregnant or has a medical condition, such as liver disease, heart disease, cancer, or diabetes.

SEVERED LIMB

A limb can be completely severed or partially severed and still attached by tissue or skin. Fingers, hands, toes, arms, or legs can be involved in these accidents.

A severed limb can often be reattached by surgery. The success of this surgery depends on how quickly the victim gets to the hospital and how well the severed part has been stored. If stored properly (see page 142), a severed limb can remain viable for up to 18 hours.

What To Look For

•A missing limb or a limb that is still attached by damaged tissue or skin

•Severe bleeding, particularly when a limb is partially severed. When a victim's limb is completely severed, blood vessels often collapse or close, limiting blood loss.

•Pain

•Shock (see page 146)

What To Do (and Not To Do)

•Check the victim's ABCs (see page 9) and treat as necessary.

•Call 911 (EMS).

•Try to stop any bleeding by applying direct pressure to the wound site. Raise the limb if it's still attached and apply a dry dressing or cloths to the wound.

•To help prevent shock, lay the victim down with legs elevated (this will increase blood flow to the heart and brain) and keep him warm with a blanket or coat (see page 147). *AVOID* moving the victim if a spinal cord injury is suspected (see page 154).

•After you're certain the victim is stable, try to locate the severed limb. No matter how small the body part, always take the following steps to store it for transport to the hospital:

> •If possible, remove debris from the severed limb. Using clean water, rinse the limb. *DO NOT* scrub it.

> •Wrap the severed limb in moist, clean cloths. Sterile gauze is a good choice.

> •Put the wrapped limb in a clean plastic bag, or wrap it in plastic wrap.

> •If possible, put the bag into a plastic bag or container filled with slush (ice mixed with water). Cooling the amputated limb will improve the chances of successful reattachment. Be sure the ice never directly touches the amputated limb.

> •Label the package with the victim's name and time of the accident.

•Check for injuries other than the severed limb. If so, treat as required.

CHECK

Airway

Breathing

Circulation

•Stay with the victim, comforting him until EMS arrive. Give the package containing the severed limb to EMS. It should always go with the victim to the hospital.

SEXUAL ASSAULT AND SEXUAL ABUSE

Sexual assault and sexual abuse can happen to men and women of all ages and from all walks of life. These crimes affect both the minds and bodies of their victims. For information on abuse of children, see Child Abuse, page 60.

You can do much to aid the victims of sexual crimes, providing help not only for their physical injuries but for their emotional ones as well. When interacting with a sexual assault victim, it's vital to convey your belief in their experience and to offer your support and understanding.

What To Look For

SEXUAL ASSAULT
•Bruising and bleeding in genital area
•Other injuries associated with assault, such as marks from strangling or kicking
•Object embedded in a body opening
•Extreme anxiety, fear, or depression
•Loss of consciousness

SEXUAL ABUSE
•Discomfort, bruising, and bleeding in genital area
•Pain when urinating
•Discomfort when sitting or walking
•Extreme fear of a person or place
•Abrupt change in behavior
•Anxiety, fear, or depression
•Sexually transmitted disease
•Pregnancy

S

What To Do (and Not To Do)

SEXUAL ASSAULT

- Check the victim's ABCs and treat as necessary (see page 9).
- Call 911 (EMS). Ask unnecessary bystanders to leave immediately.
- Provide comfort, support, and privacy. *DO NOT* leave the victim alone.
- To help prevent shock, lay the victim down with legs elevated (this will increase blood flow to the heart and brain) and keep the victim warm with a blanket or coat (see page 147). *AVOID* moving the victim if a spinal cord injury is suspected (for more details, see page 154).
- If possible, *DO NOT* allow the victim to change clothes, bathe, brush teeth, douche, urinate, or defecate. This is important for preserving potential evidence.
- The victim may want to consider taking emergency contraception, which can prevent pregnancy after unprotected sexual intercourse by stopping or delaying ovulation, stopping transport of the egg or sperm in the fallopian tubes, interfering with contraception, or stopping the fertilized egg from attaching to the uterus (by causing the lining of the uterus to shed). There are 2 types of emergency contraception:

  - The most common method of emergency contraception is the emergency contraception pill (ECP), which contains estrogen and progestin, the two hormones most commonly found in birth control pills. To be most effective, the first dose of ECP should be taken *within 72 hours* of unprotected intercourse, and the second dose taken 12 hours later. ECP is available from Planned Parenthood health centers; college, public, and women's health centers; private doctors; and some hospital emergency rooms. In some states, pharmacists can provide ECP directly.

  - A second method of emergency contraception is the intra-uterine device (IUD), which can be

CHECK

AIRWAY
BREATHING
CIRCULATION

S

inserted by a physician up to 5 days after unprotected intercourse. This option is not advisable for some women (such as those with previous pelvic inflammatory disease or with a sexually transmitted disease).

IF THERE IS BLEEDING

•Wash your hands with soap and water. Expose as little of the genital area as possible. *DO NOT* wash the wound.

•Place a sterile pad or clean cloth over the wound and apply direct, constant pressure. *DO NOT* remove blood-stained dressings; instead, place another on top, to soak up the blood. *DO NOT* apply direct pressure to an embedded object; press down firmly on either side of the injury. *DO NOT* remove the embedded object, but try to stabilize it by using bulky cloths or dressings.

•If there is severe vaginal bleeding, you may need to pack the vagina with pads or clean cloths to stop the bleeding (see Genital Injury, page 104).

•Apply a covered ice pack or cold compress to the injured area to reduce swelling.

SEXUAL ABUSE

•Offer comfort and let the victim know that you can be trusted.

•Listen carefully and take the victim seriously.

•Encourage the victim to report the abuse.

•Help the victim to find support and counseling services.

IF THE VICTIM IS PHYSICALLY INJURED OR UNCONSCIOUS

•Check the victim's ABCs and treat as necessary (see page 9).

•Call 911 (EMS).

•Attend to any physical injuries.

•To help prevent shock, lay the victim down with legs elevated (this will increase blood flow to the heart and brain) and keep the victim warm with a blanket or coat (see page 147). *AVOID* moving the

CHECK

Airway

Breathing

Circulation

S

victim if a spinal cord injury is suspected (for more details, see page 154).

•Calm the victim and wait for EMS to arrive.

SHOCK

Shock is a condition that develops when there is not enough blood or fluids traveling to the body's vital organs, such as the heart and brain. Shock can be caused by a heart problem (when the heart fails to pump blood throughout the body), severe loss of blood or other fluids, severe infection (septic shock), dehydration, burns, or damage to the nervous system (such as spinal cord injury).

We may sometimes use the word "shock" to describe an emotional state brought on by an upsetting situation. It's important not to confuse the two—emotional distress, although real, is not the same as the physiologic condition that is discussed here.

What To Look For

•Pale, cold, clammy skin (spinal or septic shock can result in hot, flushed skin)

•Sweating

SOME TYPES OF SHOCK

ANAPHYLACTIC SHOCK
Anaphylactic shock is caused by a severe allergic reaction. During this reaction, the blood vessels in the body are enlarged, causing a sudden drop in blood pressure (see Allergic Reactions, page 31).

CARDIAC SHOCK
Cardiac shock occurs when the heart cannot pump normally; this causes the blood pressure to decrease and results in not enough blood getting to the vital organs.

SEPTIC/TOXIC SHOCK
Septic or toxic shock develops when an infection in the bloodstream prevents body tissues and organs from using nutrients in the blood.

SPINAL SHOCK
A spinal shock occurs when the spinal cord is injured and can no longer regulate the blood vessels. These vessels enlarge, creating a sudden drop in blood pressure and hot, flushed skin (see Spinal Injury, page 154).

•Skin around the mouth and lips is blue (see also page 15)
•Thirst
•Nausea and vomiting
•Rapid, shallow breathing
•Rapid pulse that may become weaker
•Anxiety, restlessness
•Dizziness, lightheadedness, especially when rising
•Loss of consciousness

What To Do (and Not To Do)

•Check the victim's ABCs and treat as necessary (see page 9).
•Call 911 (EMS).
•Keep the victim warm with a blanket or coat.
•Provide first aid for the illness or injury causing the shock.

IF YOU DO NOT SUSPECT A SPINAL INJURY
•Lay the victim down with legs elevated (to increase blood flow to the heart and brain). This is called the shock position.

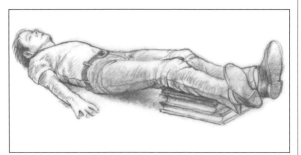

CHECK
AIRWAY
BREATHING
CIRCULATION

To prevent or reduce shock, place the victim in the shock position and then cover him with blankets or coats to keep him warm.

•If the victim is vomiting or drooling, turn him onto his left side. This is called the recovery position and will help prevent further vomiting and allow fluids to drain from his mouth (for details, see page 11).
•If the victim has breathing difficulties, raise his head and shoulders (without creating discomfort), instead of using the shock position.

IF YOU SUSPECT A SPINAL INJURY

•If the victim is vomiting or drooling, carefully log-roll him onto his left side. Support his head and neck, keep his head in line with his body, and roll the body as one unit. If possible, have three or more people help you do this. *DO NOT* move the victim unless absolutely necessary. If you must move the victim (due to an unsafe situation), see Moving a Spinal Injury Victim, page 156.

SMOKE INHALATION

Smoke from any type of fire can contain poisonous substances. When the smoke is inhaled, the victim's airways can be injured and breathing may become difficult.

By quickly removing the victim from the smoke's source and monitoring the victim's ABCs—airway, breathing, and circulation (pulse)—you can help prevent or reduce the damage from smoke inhalation.

What To Look For
•Coughing
•Breath has a smoky or chemical smell
•Black deposits in nose and mouth
•Burned nose hairs
•Difficulty breathing
•Loss of consciousness

What To Do (and Not To Do)
•Immediately move the victim to fresh air away from the source of the smoke. Take care to ensure that you don't become a victim yourself (for details, see page 24).
•Check the victim's ABCs and treat as necessary (see page 9).
•Call 911 (EMS).
•Loosen any tight clothing, particularly around the victim's neck.
•Turn the victim onto his left side. This is called the recovery position and will prevent vomiting

CHECK

Airway

Breathing

Circulation

and allow fluids to drain from his mouth (for details, see page 11).

•If the victim is having trouble breathing, gently raise his head and shoulders, or place him in a sitting position.

•Check the victim for any burns and treat as required (see Thermal Burns, page 164).

SNAKE BITES

There are many snakes in the United States but only two types—pit vipers and coral snakes—are poisonous. Pit vipers, including rattlesnakes, copperheads, and cottonmouths, affect the circulatory system; coral snakes affect the nervous system.

Certain defining features distinguish pit vipers and coral snakes from nonpoisonous snakes (see page 150). Local poison control centers are expert in helping you tell the difference.

Emergency medical care is essential so that the victim can be given antivenin (a fluid that contains antibodies that counteract the venom). Until then, you can calm the victim, monitor his vital signs, and help to slow down the spread of venom throughout the body.

What To Look For

PIT VIPERS
•One or two small puncture wounds in the skin
•Severe pain and burning at the site of the bite
•Sudden, rapid swelling in the affected area
•Blood blisters and discoloration around the bite
•Shock (see page 146)

CORAL SNAKES
•Minor pain at site
•Drowsiness
•Staggering
•Difficulty speaking
•Vision problems

DISTINGUISHING PIT VIPERS AND CORAL SNAKES

PIT VIPER FEATURES
- Flat, triangular head
- Vertical eyes (shaped like those of a cat)
- Pits between eyes and nostrils
- Single row (instead of a double row) of plates on the underside of the tail

CORAL SNAKE FEATURES
- Black snout
- Colorful body—alternating bands of red, yellow, and black (every other band is yellow)
- Round eyes

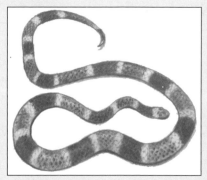

Coral snake

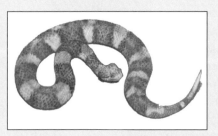

Broad-banded copperhead snake, a type of pit viper.

- Sweating
- Drooling
- Nausea
- Seizures

NONPOISONOUS SNAKES
- Horseshoe shape of toothmarks on skin
- Mild pain and swelling

CHECK

AIRWAY

BREATHING

CIRCULATION

What To Do (and Not To Do)

IF THE VICTIM HAS BEEN BITTEN BY A POISONOUS SNAKE
- Check the victim's ABCs and treat as necessary (see page 9).
- Call 911 (EMS). If possible, inform them which type of snake has bitten the victim so an antivenin can be prepared.

S

•Remove all jewelry from the injured area.

•Move the victim (by carrying or gently walking with him) and anyone else away from the snake.

•Lay the victim down and keep him still to help slow down the spread of venom. If you can, immobilize an affected limb with a splint (see page 52).

•Gently wash the bite area with soap and water. *DO NOT* apply an ice pack to the wound. *DO NOT* cut the victim's skin or attempt to extract the venom with your mouth. Consider using a snake bite suction kit if one is available, and you have been trained to use it.

•Place the bitten area below the level of the victim's heart, if possible.

•If shock develops, lay the victim down with legs elevated (to increase blood flow to the heart and brain). This is called the shock position (see page 147). If you suspect a spinal injury, *DO NOT* elevate the bitten area or move the victim into the shock position, and *DO NOT* elevate a leg above the level of the victim's heart if the leg has been bitten. Cover the victim with blankets or coats to keep him warm.

•If the victim is vomiting or drooling, turn him onto his left side. This is called the recovery position and will help prevent vomiting and allow fluids to drain from his mouth (see page 11). If you suspect a spinal cord injury, carefully log-roll him onto his left side, supporting his head and neck and always keeping his head in line with his body. If possible, have three or more people help you do this (see page 155).

•*DO NOT* give the victim any food or drink.

•Transport only dead snakes to the hospital, in a sealed container.

IF VICTIM HAS BEEN BITTEN BY A NONPOISONOUS SNAKE

•Gently wash the snake bite with soap and water.

•Cover with a clean, dry dressing.

•Seek medical care and have the victim obtain a tetanus booster immunization if necessary.

S

BLACK WIDOW SPIDER
- Black, brown, or gray
- Round abdomen with red or yellow spots (sometimes in the shape of an hourglass) or white spots or bands

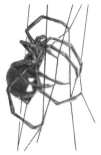

BROWN RECLUSE SPIDER
- Light to dark brown with darker legs
- Violin shape on back

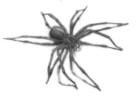

TARANTULA
- Very large
- Hairy

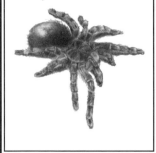

SPIDER BITES

While many spiders can bite, only two types—black widow spiders and brown recluse spiders—inject venom that is dangerous and potentially life-threatening to humans. Although not life-threatening, tarantula bites can cause local, and sometimes serious, reactions.

Recognizing the type of spider that has bitten the victim is important for determining the right treatment. Antivenin (a fluid that contains antibodies that counteract the venom) is available for black widow spider bites, although it's usually given only to children less than 5 years of age, pregnant women, the elderly, or victims with severe bites. There is no antivenin for brown recluse or other spider bites.

Remember that your local poison control center is an invaluable source for advice on handling spider bites.

What To Look For

BLACK WIDOW SPIDER
- Symptoms appear 1 to 24 hours after the bite
- Numbness at the bite site
- Skin rash
- Severe pain and muscle spasms
- Severe abdominal cramps
- Dizziness
- Sweating
- Nausea and vomiting
- Tightness in the chest
- Difficulty breathing

BROWN RECLUSE SPIDER
- Symptoms begin to appear within a few hours
- Pain at the bite site
- Swelling and tenderness
- Rash
- Blisters that can form painful ulcers (craters)

S

- Fever
- Weakness
- Stomach and joint pain
- Nausea and vomiting

TARANTULA
- Mild pain to deep throbbing pain
- Itching
- Hives
- Sores that may take some time to heal

What To Do (and Not To Do)
- Check the victim's ABCs and treat as necessary (see page 9).

IF THE VICTIM HAS BEEN BITTEN BY A BLACK WIDOW, BROWN RECLUSE, OR TARANTULA SPIDER
- Seek immediate medical care or go to the emergency room.
- Try to identify which type of spider has bitten the victim, and tell the doctor so an antivenin can be prepared, if possible. If you can kill the spider without endangering yourself, do so and take it to the hospital along with the victim.
- If the victim is having trouble breathing, place him in a sitting position.
- If the victim vomits, turn him onto his left side. This is called the recovery position and will prevent further vomiting and allow fluids to drain from his mouth (see page 11). If you suspect a spinal cord injury, carefully log-roll him onto his left side, supporting his head and neck and always keeping his head in line with his body. If possible, have three or more people help you do this (see page 155).

IF THE VICTIM HAS BEEN BITTEN BY A NONPOISONOUS SPIDER
- Gently wash the bite with soap and water.
- Cover with a clean, dry dressing.
- Seek medical care if the bite becomes red, tender, or swollen.

CHECK

Airway
Breathing
Circulation

SPINAL INJURY

The spine is a column of small bones (called vertebrae) that extends from the base of the skull to the tailbone. These vertebrae surround and protect the spinal cord, a thick cord of nerves that relays messages from the brain to the rest of the body. A spinal injury may only damage the vertebrae (for example, a fracture) or it may damage the spinal cord itself, potentially resulting in the permanent loss of feeling or in paralysis in the area below the injury.

Falls, diving accidents, and motor vehicle collisions are just some of the ways a victim can suffer a spinal injury.

Whenever you encounter a victim who is unconscious or who has a head, neck, or back injury, assume that a spinal injury has occurred. You have an important role to play in preventing further damage to the spine or spinal cord.

What To Look For
•Symptoms appearing almost immediately after the injury has occurred
•Numbness or tingling
•Weakness
•Paralysis
•Hot, flushed skin
•Weak pulse
•Difficulty breathing
•Pain from injury to surrounding nerves
•Severe pain in the back or neck
•Loss of bladder or bowel control

What To Do (and Not To Do)
•Check the victim's ABCs and treat as necessary (see page 9). If the victim is not lying on his back and requires rescue breathing or CPR, gently log-roll him onto his back. Support his head and neck, and roll the body as one unit. If possible, have three or more people help you do this. To open the vic-

S

CHECK

AIRWAY

BREATHING

CIRCULATION

tim's airway, *DO NOT* move the head or neck. Try lifting the chin without tilting his head back. If the breaths don't go in, gently tilt the head back until they do.

•Call 911 (EMS).

•Keep the victim still. *DO NOT* move the victim unless absolutely necessary (see Moving a Spinal Injury Victim, page 156). If the victim is wearing a motorcycle or bicycle helmet, *DO NOT* try to remove it.

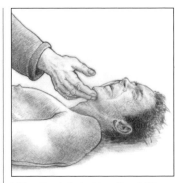
Lifting the victim's chin without tilting the head back.

•Immobilize the victim's spine by padding the head, neck, and back with pillows or bulky towels. Support those with any available heavier objects such as bricks or books.

•Check the victim for other injuries, and treat as required.

•Cover the victim with blankets or coats to keep him warm and help prevent shock. *DO NOT* move the victim into the shock position—lying down with legs elevated.

•If the victim vomits, carefully log-roll him onto his left side. Support his head and neck, keep his head in line with his body, and roll his body as one unit. If possible, have three or more people help you do this.

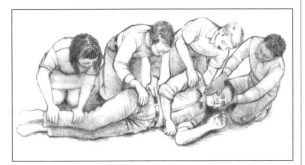
When a victim with a spinal injury is vomiting, carefully log-roll him onto his left side.

S

MOVING A SPINAL INJURY VICTIM

DO NOT move a victim with a spinal injury unless the situation is dangerous and life-threatening. If you must move the victim, always follow these ground rules:
• Move the victim in the position you found him, face up, face down, or lying on his side.
• Move the body in one smooth motion, always keeping the victim's head in line with his body.
• When possible, have other people help you move the victim.
• *DO NOT* rotate the head, neck, shoulder, or pelvis.
• *DO NOT* move a victim sideways.

IF YOU ARE ALONE, DRAG THE VICTIM, USING HIS CLOTHES
• Grab hold of the victim's clothes around his shoulders, using your forearms to stabilize his head. Unbutton any clothing at the neck that might choke the victim.
• Bend your knees while you pull, keeping your weight low to the ground.
• Pull backward in a smooth motion until the victim is clear of the area.

IF OTHERS CAN ASSIST, USE THE LOG-ROLL
• Find a board or other large, rigid surface, such as a door, to carry the victim. If nothing is available, use your hands.
• Place yourself at the victim's head so you can make sure the head and body move as one unit.
• Position the board close to the victim so you can slide it under his back.
• Ask the others to place their hands on the far side of the victim. Then, in one motion, carefully log-roll the victim onto the board. *DO NOT* twist the victim's head, neck, shoulder, or back.
• Place rolled towels or blankets around the victim's head to immobilize it, and secure them in place with a tie.
• Secure the victim to the board with long ties, or hold the victim in place with your hands. Gently lift the board, keeping the victim's head and body in line.

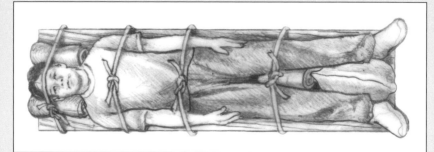

Victim of a spinal injury secured on a board.

SPLINTERS

See Puncture Wounds, page 133

STINGS

See Insect Stings, page 118; Marine Animal Bites and Stings, page 121; and Scorpion Stings, page 137

STRAINS AND SPRAINS

During the course of our busy, active lives, injuries to muscles and joints are all too common.

In the case of strains, muscles are stretched or torn, but ligaments remain undamaged. Sprains, on the other hand, involve torn or stretched joints with damage to ligaments and joint capsules (coverings).

In most strains and sprains, the use of RICE (rest, ice, compression, and elevation, see page 158) can help speed recovery time and return the victim to his regular activities. More severe injuries, such as joint dislocations, will take longer to heal.

What To Look For

STRAINS
•Pain, tenderness, and stiffness at the site of injury
•Indentation or bump
•Weakness and loss of function in limb

SPRAINS
•Pain, tenderness, and swelling at injury site
•Bruising
•Unstable joint
•Weakness and loss of function in limb

S

RICE: REST, ICE, COMPRESSION, ELEVATION

•**Rest** the victim in a comfortable position, either sitting up or lying down.

•**Ice**—Apply an ice pack to the injured muscle and secure with an elastic bandage. The injury should be iced for 20 to 30 minutes (but no longer), every 2 to 3 hours for 24 to 48 hours. Be sure not to stop the icing process too soon.

•**Compression**—Provide compression to the injury by wrapping it with an elastic bandage. Begin bandaging below the injury and wrap upwards using relatively tight pressure. Gradually reduce the pressure as you finish wrapping above the injury. Be sure not to wrap too tightly. The victim should wear the bandage continuously for 18 to 24 hours. The bandage should be loosened if the victim finds it uncomfortable.

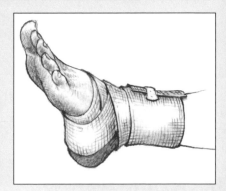

Compression bandage on an injured ankle.

•**Elevation**—Elevate the injured part above the victim's heart (if possible) during icing and compression.

What To Do (and Not To Do)

MUSCLE STRAINS AND MILD SPRAINS

•Start the RICE procedure right away (see above).

•Apply heat after 48 to 72 hours.

•Give the victim ibuprofen or, if an adult, aspirin to relieve the pain and inflammation of the muscle injury.

•If injury is severe or doesn't improve, seek medical assistance.

SEVERE SPRAIN

•If necessary, remove or cut away clothing around the injury. Remove rings and constricting jewelry as well.

•Check for pain, swelling, and tenderness at the injury site. Make every effort not to move the injured area.

•Immobilize the injury by padding it with pillows and towels. If EMS are not nearby and you must get the victim to the hospital, you should splint the injured limb (see page 52).

•Place an ice pack (wrapped in a cloth) or a cold compress on the injured area to ease pain and swelling. If it's not too painful for the victim, elevate the injury.

•To help prevent shock, lay the victim down with legs elevated (this will increase blood flow to the heart and brain) and keep him warm with a blanket or coat (see page 147). *AVOID* moving the victim if a spinal cord injury is suspected (for more details, see page 154).

•Call 911 (EMS) or seek immediate medical attention.

STROKE

A stroke, or "brain attack," occurs when the blood supply to the brain is reduced or completely blocked, depriving the brain of all-important oxygen.

There are two main types of strokes:

•*Hemorrhagic stroke*—a blood vessel in the brain leaks or bursts. Blood fills the surrounding brain tissue and damages it. Brain cells beyond the leak don't receive blood and are damaged as well.

•*Ischemic stroke*—a blood clot or other material plugs a blood vessel in the brain.

The effects of a stroke depend on how much of the brain and which area was damaged. Although these effects can be devastating, we know that early recognition and treatment of stroke can reduce brain damage and disability. In fact, research has shown that, in some ischemic strokes, medication can help prevent brain damage if given within 3 hours of the onset of symptoms. Therefore, early recognition is crucial to the successful treatment of stroke.

You can play a positive, proactive role by becoming familiar with the signs of stroke and acting quickly when they arise.

FOR MORE INFORMATION...

The National Institute of Neurological Disorders and Stroke (NINDS) can provide a wealth of information on neurologic disorders, including stroke. See page 251.

What To Look For
•Sudden numbness or weakness of face, arm, or leg, especially on one side of the body
•Sudden confusion, trouble speaking, or trouble understanding speech
•Sudden trouble seeing in one or both eyes
•Sudden trouble walking, dizziness, loss of balance or coordination
•Sudden severe headache with no known cause

What To Do (and Not To Do)
•Check the victim's ABCs and treat as necessary (see page 9).
•Call 911 (EMS) or take the victim to the emergency room.
•Place the victim in a comfortable position.
•If the victim vomits or loses consciousness, turn him on his left side. This is called the recovery position and will prevent further vomiting and allow fluids to drain from his mouth (see page 11).
•*DO NOT* give the victim food or drink.
•Continue to monitor the victim's ABCs until EMS arrive.

CHECK

AIRWAY
BREATHING
CIRCULATION

FOR MORE INFORMATION...

Many organizations, such as the National Mental Health Association, offer information and referrals on mental health. See page 253.

SUICIDAL THREATS OR BEHAVIOR

Suicide, the act of taking one's own life, claims victims of all ages and from all walks of life. Suicide is not necessarily a sign of mental illness; it can also result from other conditions and situations such as extreme grief over the loss of a loved one, as well as substance abuse or severe financial problems.

Whenever you observe the warning signs of suicide, take them seriously and ensure that the victim receives immediate professional help. Saved from suicide, most people can then go on to lead productive lives.

What To Look For
•Threat or talk of suicide
•Depression—feelings of overwhelming sadness, guilt, worthlessness, hopelessness

•Agitation, mood swings, changes in personality, and difficulty sleeping
•Prolonged withdrawal from people and activities
•Self-destructive, risky behavior such as reckless driving or unsafe sex
•Delusions or hallucinations
•Saying goodbye to friends and family, suddenly preparing a will or making arrangements for a funeral

What To Do (and Not To Do)

•Always take seriously any talk or threats of suicide.
•Ask the person directly about his intentions if he doesn't overtly talk of suicide, but you suspect he is thinking about it.
•Listen closely to the person and express your concern and support. *DO NOT* leave the person alone. Stay with him until professional help arrives.
•Help the person to seek professional help immediately. Call 911 (EMS) if necessary.
•Provide ongoing support to the person.

SUNBURN

Sunburn is caused by overexposure to the sun's ultraviolet (UV) rays. Sun lamps and tanning beds can be equally damaging.

Damage usually results in superficial burns (minor damage to the top layer of skin). More severe burns can be partial thickness (skin is damaged but its full depth is not completely destroyed, see page 54).

When it comes to the initial steps of first aid, sunburn is no different from other burns—stop the burning process and cool the burn.

What To Look For

•Redness and itching
•Tenderness
•Swelling
•Blisters

S

SUNBURN PREVENTION POINTERS

You can take a variety of steps in order to prevent sunburn.

•Stay out of the sun when its rays are strongest—between 10 AM and 3 PM—and when the UV index is high. Be aware that the sun's harmful rays can penetrate clouds, water, and some fabrics.

•Always use sunscreen or sunblock, whether you're at the beach, in the garden, or on the ski slopes. Choose a broad-spectrum sunscreen with a sun protection factor (SPF) of at least 15. Apply the sunscreen liberally to all exposed areas at least 15 to 30 minutes before going out. Be sure your children use sunscreen regularly. *DO NOT* use sunscreen on infants under 6 months of age (their bodies can't handle the sunscreen's chemicals). Instead, keep your baby in the shade and dress him in proper clothing and a hat (see below).

•Wear a hat, ideally one with at least a 3-inch brim or with flaps that hang down from all sides.

•Don't forget about sunglasses, even for young children. Wrap-around models with large frames are the best choice. To protect you, sunglasses must block 99% to 100% of UVA and UVB radiation. Check the label to be sure.

•Whenever possible, wear long-sleeved shirts and long pants or skirts when in the sun. Choose fabrics with a tight weave.

What To Do (and Not To Do)

•Get the victim out of the sun or other source of UV rays.

•Cool the burn by placing the injured area under cool water. Alternatively, you can apply cold compresses to the burn area or the victim can take frequent, cool showers.

•To reduce inflammation, apply lotions (such as aloe vera gel), a sunburn relief spray, or over-the-counter hydrocortisone cream to the affected area.

•Give the victim plenty of cool water to drink.

•Acetaminophen or ibuprofen or, if an adult, aspirin, can help relieve the victim's pain.

•*DO NOT* break blisters if they develop. If the blisters pop on their own, wash the area with an antibacterial soap and cover with a clean, dry dressing. Seek medical care.

IF THE SUNBURN IS SEVERE

•Stop the burning process and cool the burn (as above).

•Cover the burn area with a clean, dry dressing and, if possible, elevate it.

•Seek medical attention. The doctor may give the victim a prescription ointment or other necessary medication.

•Watch for signs of infection (pain, tenderness, pus, or red streaks).

TEETH PAIN AND INJURY

See Dental Pain and Injuries, page 78

TETANUS

Tetanus, also known as lockjaw, is caused when a bacterium found in rust, soil, and animal feces enters a wound or cut of a nonimmunized person. This bacterium produces a poison that travels through the nervous system to the brain, causing spasms in the back, arms, legs, and jaw.

In most cases, tetanus is a serious, life-threatening condition that does not respond to treatment. That's why prevention is so important. A tetanus vaccine, in use for more than 50 years, is highly effective. But an initial vaccine *MUST* be followed up by boosters at 5- to 10-year intervals to maintain protection against tetanus. Keep track of your family's immunization status, and be sure to get boosters as recommended by your doctor.

In cases of animal bites or cuts (particularly deep puncture wounds), it is vital to check a victim's tetanus immunization status. A tetanus shot will be required if

•The victim has never been immunized against tetanus.

•The victim has not received a booster in the last 10 years or within 5 years if the wound is dirty, deep, or infected.

See also Cat, Dog, and Other Animal Bites (page 56), Cuts (Lacerations) (page 74), and Puncture Wounds (page 133).

T–N

THERMAL BURNS

Thermal burns can be caused by both wet heat, such as steam or hot liquid, or dry heat (for example, from a hot stove or flames).

Your response to a thermal burn injury depends on the depth of the burn, as well as its location and size. But no matter what, stopping the burning process and cooling the burn is your first priority.

What To Look For

SUPERFICIAL BURNS (MINOR DAMAGE TO THE TOP LAYER OF SKIN)
•Redness
•Mild swelling and pain

PARTIAL-THICKNESS BURNS (SKIN IS DAMAGED BUT ITS FULL DEPTH IS NOT COMPLETELY DESTROYED)
•Raw appearance
•Severe swelling and pain
•Blisters
•Fluid seeping from burn area

FULL-THICKNESS BURNS (FULL DEPTH OF SKIN, HAIR FOLLICLES, MUSCLES, NERVES, BONES, AND INTERNAL ORGANS ARE DAMAGED OR DESTROYED)
•Skin looks gray, waxy, leathery, or charred
•No pain

What To Do (and Not To Do)

•Stop the burning immediately. Put out any flames by dousing the victim with water or smothering flames with a blanket.
•Cool the burn by placing the injured area under cool water. If water isn't available, a cool drink, such as a soft drink or iced tea, will do. If you can't immerse the injured area in water or liquid, use wet, cool towels. Replace the towels frequently to maintain the cool temperature.

•Remove all hot or burned clothes and jewelry. Don't pull off clothing that is stuck to the skin. Cut off as much as you can instead.
•Check the size, location, and depth of the burn injury and treat as below.
•Check the victim's tetanus immunization status. If not up to date, he may require a tetanus shot.

SIZE AND LOCATION

If any depth of burn covers a large area (more than 15% of an adult's body or more than 10% of a child's body) or is on the face, hands, feet, or genitals, do the following:
•Check the victim's ABCs (see page 9) and treat as necessary.
•Call 911 (EMS).
•Continue to cool the burn area until EMS arrive.
•To help prevent shock, lay the victim down with legs elevated (this will increase blood flow to the heart and brain) (see page 147). *AVOID* moving the victim if a spinal cord injury is suspected (see page 154).
•If possible, elevate the burn area.

DEPTH

Superficial Burn

•Continue cooling the victim's burn for at least 10 minutes.
•Give the victim ibuprofen or, if an adult, aspirin to relieve pain and inflammation.
•First aid ointments may be applied and may relieve symptoms and prevent infection. *DO NOT* apply butter or oil-based home remedies.
•Cover with a clean, dry gauze dressing. *DO NOT* use a wet or plastic dressing, or fluffy material.

PARTIAL-THICKNESS BURN

Follow the recommendations for superficial burn (see above), and in addition
•*DO NOT* burst any blister that may form.
•Seek medical attention.

CHECK

Airway

Breathing

Circulation

SUNBURNS

Sunburns are superficial burns that develop after overexposure to the sun's UV rays. They usually differ from other thermal burns, developing over a longer period of time. For more information on sunburn, see page 161.

T-N

> **CHECK**
>
> Airway
>
> Breathing
>
> Circulation

> **PREVENTION POINTERS**
>
> You can stay clear of ticks with a few simple steps. First, find out whether your area has disease-carrying ticks. If it does, be sure to wear appropriate clothing, covering as much skin as possible, and keep away from tall grass and dense woods, where ticks may be hiding. Then, perform periodic total body checks for ticks during and after your outdoor activities.

Deer ticks, particularly in the nymph stage, are very small (bottom of figure; ticks are also shown enlarged, in the box, for easier identification). They expand to 5 to 7 times in size after feeding on a victim's body.

FULL-THICKNESS BURN

- Check the victim's ABCs and treat as necessary (see page 9).
- Call 911 (EMS).
- Continue to cool the burn area until EMS arrive.
- Cover with a clean, dry gauze dressing. *DO NOT* use a wet or plastic dressing or fluffy material. *DO NOT* touch the burn area.
- If possible, elevate the burn area.

TICK BITES

Ticks, a close relative of spiders, are small, eight-legged creatures found on shrubs, trees, sand dunes, or other animals. They burrow into the skin of humans and animals and live off the blood of their host. Although their bites are almost always painless, several types of tick can pass on serious diseases, such as Lyme disease or Rocky Mountain spotted fever.

By recognizing a tick and removing it—both promptly and properly—you can help keep a victim free of the serious diseases that are carried by some ticks.

What To Look For

- Tick, on or burrowing into, skin
- Circular rash at bite site
- Swelling and itching

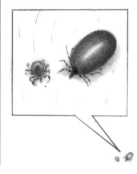

What To Do (and Not To Do)

•If you notice the tick crawling on the victim's skin, carefully brush it off. *DO NOT* crush it between your fingers. Step on it with your shoes or crush it between two rocks.

•If the tick has become embedded in the skin, use tweezers to remove it. Your goal is to remove the entire tick intact below its mouthpiece. To do this, grasp the tick close to the skin surface and pull away with steady pressure. *DO NOT* twist or forcefully tug on the tick and *DO NOT* try to remove it with a burned match, petroleum jelly, or nail polish. A tick removed within 6 hours of attachment will usually not have time to transmit disease.

•Once the tick has been removed, wash the bite site with soap and water. Apply a cold compress or covered ice pack to reduce pain and swelling. Later, pat on calamine lotion to relieve itching.

•If possible, save the tick in a jar for medical personnel to inspect.

•Check the victim's tetanus immunization status. If not up to date, he may require a tetanus shot.

•If the tick has been properly removed, it is usually not necessary to see a doctor. However, you should seek immediate medical care if the following symptoms occur:

  •A new rash

  •High fever

  •Headache

  •Nerve and joint swelling and pain

Some symptoms can occur *weeks after* a tick bite.

IF YOU CAN'T REMOVE THE ENTIRE TICK FROM THE VICTIM

•Seek immediate medical attention.

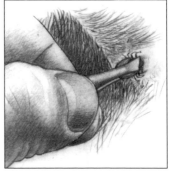

Removing a tick that is embedded in the skin.

UNCONSCIOUSNESS

Unconsciousness occurs when the normal functions of the brain are interrupted due to illness or injury, including head injury, stroke, heart attack, shock, poisoning, low blood sugar (hypoglycemia), low blood oxygen, alcohol or drug overdose, and severe allergic reaction.

When you encounter an unconscious victim, the most important step is to open the airway, check breathing and pulse, and give CPR or rescue breathing, if necessary.

What To Look For
- Unresponsiveness
- Difficulty breathing
- Large or small pupils
- Fever
- Evidence of drug abuse, such as empty bottles or needle tracks on the victim's arms or legs
- Head injury
- Exposure to carbon monoxide from space heaters or other appliances
- Medical identification bracelet (check particularly for diabetes)

What To Do (and Not To Do)
- Check the victim's ABCs and treat as necessary (see page 9).
- Call 911 (EMS).
- If the victim has diabetes, place sugar under his tongue.
- Always assume that an unconscious victim has a spinal injury.
- If the victim is not lying on his back and requires rescue breathing or CPR, gently log-roll him onto his back. Support his head and neck and roll the body as one unit. If possible, have three or more people help you do this. To open the victim's airway, *DO NOT* move the head or neck. Try lifting the chin without tilting the head back. If the

---

CHECK

A IRWAY

B REATHING

C IRCULATION

T–Z

breaths don't go in, gently tilt the head back until they do (see Spinal Injury, page 154).

•Keep the victim still. *DO NOT* move the victim unless absolutely necessary (see Moving a Spinal Injury Victim, page 156).

•Check the victim for other injuries and treat as required.

•Cover the victim with blankets or coats to keep him warm and help prevent shock. *DO NOT* move the victim into the shock position (lying down with legs elevated).

•If the victim vomits, carefully log-roll him onto his left side. Support his head and neck and roll the body as one unit. If possible, have three or more people help you do this (see page 172).

VAGINAL BLEEDING

Bleeding from the vagina not related to menstruation may be a sign of vaginal injury from a foreign object (see also Genital Injury, page 104), illness, or a complication of pregnancy, such as miscarriage.

Whenever nonmenstrual blood is coming from the vagina, seek emergency medical care. You can help the victim by providing dressings to absorb the blood and taking steps to prevent or minimize shock.

What To Look For
•Vaginal bleeding not related to menstruation
•Abdominal pain
•Contractions of the uterus
•Use of medications, such as blood thinners
•Indications of pregnancy
•Lightheadedness (if heavy bleeding)
•Shock (see page 154)

What To Do (and Not To Do)
•Check the victim's ABCs and treat as necessary (see page 9).
•Call EMS (911) or seek medical care.

CHECK

AIRWAY

BREATHING

CIRCULATION

T-Z

•Place a pad or dressing over the vaginal opening to absorb blood. *DO NOT* remove a foreign object that is in the vagina; stabilize it in place with bulky dressings.

•If there is severe vaginal bleeding, you may need to pack the vagina with pads or clean cloths to stop the bleeding.

•Vomiting can happen at any time, so keep a container, such as a pail or pot, and a damp cloth nearby.

•Lay the victim on her left side—this is called the recovery position. It will help prevent further vomiting and allow fluids to drain from her mouth (see page 171). If the victim is pregnant, it will also reduce the pressure from the fetus on her circulatory system. If you suspect a spinal injury, carefully log-roll the victim onto her left side, supporting her head and neck and keeping her head in line with her body. If possible, have three or more people help you do this (see page 172).

•To help prevent shock, lay the victim down with legs elevated (this will increase blood flow to the heart and brain) and keep her warm with a blanket or coat (see page 147). *AVOID* moving the victim if a spinal injury is suspected (see page 154).

•*AVOID* giving the victim food or drink.

•Calm the victim and stay with her until EMS arrive.

VOMITING

Vomiting can be a sign of a minor illness, such as the flu, or the result of consuming too much alcohol. In these cases, it will resolve in a day or two. In other cases, vomiting can signal a more serious condition or injury, including diabetic emergencies, head injury, heart attack, food poisoning, and spider or snake bites.

Keep an eye on a victim who is vomiting, and if serious signs develop (see page 171), be prepared to seek medical attention.

T-Z

What To Look For

•Vomit that looks like coffee grounds or that contains bright, red blood

•Diarrhea

•Dehydration—dry mouth, cracked lips, severe thirst, no urination

•Abdominal cramps

•Abdominal bloating

•Head injury

•Fever

What To Do (and Not To Do)

•Have the victim lie down in the recovery position.

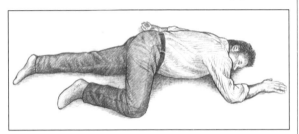

Recovery position for a victim who is vomiting.

•Give the victim plenty of fluids such as water, diluted juice, or ice chips. *AVOID* giving carbonated drinks or drinks containing caffeine or alcohol (see Dehydration, page 77).

•*DO NOT* give the victim food until vomiting has ceased for at least several hours and he is hungry.

•*DO NOT* give the victim any medication unless instructed by a doctor.

•The victim should avoid dairy products for the first 24 hours after vomiting has stopped.

IF THE VICTIM IS UNCONSCIOUS AND VOMITING

•Carefully log-roll him onto his left side. Support his head and neck, keep his head in line with his body, and roll the body as one unit. If possible, have three or more people help you do this (see page 172).

T–Z

Log-rolling the victim onto his left side.

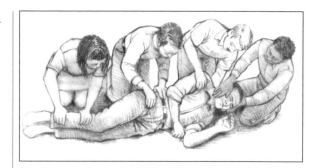

Seek medical attention if
• Diarrhea accompanies vomiting
• Vomiting is severe, forceful, or contains blood (appearance of coffee grounds)
• Victim shows signs of dehydration
• Abdominal pain is present and persistent
• Victim has suffered a head injury or is unconscious

ZIPPER INJURY

It's possible for skin to get stuck in zipper teeth while opening or closing zippers. In fact, it's not uncommon for the penis and foreskin to get caught in pant zippers. While not usually serious, a zipper injury can be painful and sometimes embarrassing for the victim. Always respect the victim's privacy, use caution when attempting to free skin from a zipper and, if necessary, seek medical care.

What To Look For
• Skin caught in the zipper
• Pain
• Swelling
• Agitation

What To Do (and Not To Do)
• Take the victim to a private place if genitalia are involved.
• *DO NOT* pull the skin free from the zipper. Cut through the zipper at the bottom so that the teeth of the zipper open.
• Seek medical attention as needed.

PLAYING IT SAFE

Much of this book is about emergencies and how to respond to them. Equally important are the many ways you can prevent serious injury or illness. Whether you're at home, in the backyard, or at work, whether you're cooking, playing, driving, or hiking, there's plenty you can do to prevent emergencies from happening and to keep everyone in your entire family happy, healthy, and safe for now and in the future.

PLAYING IT SAFE AT HOME

CARBON MONOXIDE AND RADON: SILENT KILLERS

You may often wonder about the effect of outdoor air pollution on you and your family. But you should also consider the potential for indoor pollution from carbon monoxide (CO) and radon.

Both CO and radon are toxic gases that can build up in your home and be extremely hazardous to your health. What's more, you can't see, taste or smell these gases, so many victims are unaware of their presence. The good news is that there are many steps you can take to prevent CO and radon poisoning in your home.

Carbon Monoxide

Carbon monoxide (CO) is produced by appliances or heaters that burn gas, oil, wood, propane, or kerosene. Normally, CO will dissipate and not pose a problem. However, if levels get too high, a person can be poisoned due to lack of oxygen. Left untreated, CO poisoning is life-threatening.

HOW YOU CAN PREVENT CO POISONING

Carbon Monoxide Alarms

CO alarms (also called detectors or monitors) will sound when dangerous levels of the gas are pre-

SOURCES OF CARBON MONOXIDE

A build up of CO levels can be caused by
• Malfunctioning appliances
• Clogged chimney or vent in a stove, furnace, or fireplace
• Using a nonelectric space heater in an enclosed area
• Running the car in a garage attached to the house
• Using a charcoal grill in the house or a close-by area
• Riding in the enclosed back of a pickup truck.

sent. Since you can't detect CO otherwise (remember, you can't see, taste, or smell it), CO alarms are the only way to be warned of the gas's presence. Tips for using alarms are to

•Install CO alarms on each level of your home, particularly near bedrooms. An electric model with a battery pack (in case the power goes out) is the best choice. Make sure the alarm meets with the requirements of the Underwriters Laboratories (UL) standard 2034.

•Test all your alarms at least once a month to ensure that they're in good working order.

•Replace your alarms according to the manufacturer's recommendations. Most CO alarms need to be replaced every 2 to 5 years.

Appliances and Heaters in Your Home

•Have all appliances and heaters in your home installed properly. In most cases, you should have a qualified professional do the installation to ensure adequate venting and air supply.

•Regularly maintain your appliances and heaters. On an annual basis, have a qualified service technician check and, when necessary, service your central and room-heating appliances, gas water heaters, and gas dryers. Be sure that all chimneys and flues are inspected for blockages, loose connections, and corrosion.

Watch for Signs and Symptoms of CO Poisoning

Look for symptoms that come and go, that worsen when you're in a particular area of your home, or that also appear in other family members and pets (see also page 55).

If you think anyone in your home is suffering from CO poisoning, act quickly to remove yourself and others from the area immediately and make sure to call 911 (EMS).

Radon

Radon is produced by the natural breakdown of uranium in rock, soil, and water. Usually, this gas

---

PREVENTING CO POISONING: WHAT NOT TO DO

•*DO NOT* use a charcoal or gas barbecue inside your home or in a closed space such as a garage or tent.

•*DO NOT* use gas or kerosene space heaters in poorly ventilated rooms. These heaters should never be left on overnight or in a room you're sleeping or resting in.

•*DO NOT* run the car in an attached garage or even while you're sitting in the car for an extended period outside.

•*DO NOT* allow people to sit in the enclosed back of a pickup truck.

moves up from the ground and into the air, where it can seep through cracks and holes in foundations, floors, and walls. The radon then becomes trapped in your home. Other less common sources of radon include well water and building materials.

Any home can have a radon problem—old or new, drafty or well-sealed—even homes without basements. Exposure to this gas may not immediately produce health problems. However, over prolonged periods, high levels of radon are believed to be associated with cancer. In fact, radon is believed to be second only to smoking as the leading cause of lung cancer.

HOW YOU CAN PREVENT OR REDUCE YOUR EXPOSURE TO RADON

Test Your Home for Radon

Testing is the only way to tell whether radon is present in your home. It's quick, easy, and inexpensive. Kits are available in hardware stores or other retail outlets. Make sure the kit you buy meets Environmental Protection Agency (EPA) requirements or has been certified by your state.

There are two ways to test for radon:

•Short-terms tests that remain in your house for 2 to 90 days. The period depends on the type of kit you purchase.

•Long-term tests that remain in your home for more than 90 days. These tests take longer but will provide a better indication of year-round radon levels in your home.

Always follow the manufacturer's instructions for performing the test. The amount of radon is measured in picocuries per liter of air (pCi/L) or Working Levels (WL). See EPA Guidelines for Radon Testing, page 176.

Lowering Radon Levels in Your Home

There are many ways to reduce radon levels in your home—from sealing cracks in floors and walls to installing simple systems of fans and pipes that

GET THE FACTS ON RADON

The Environment Protection Agency (EPA) has extensive information on radon and how to reduce levels in your home. By calling the EPA's National Radon Hotline or visiting its Web site, you can obtain the right information and a range of useful publications. See page 255 for contact details.

EPA GUIDELINES FOR RADON TESTING

•Take a short-term test first. If your result is 4 pCi/L or higher (0.02 WL or higher), you could have a radon problem. Do another follow-up test to confirm the results.

•Follow up with a long-term test or another short-term test. The higher your first result, the sooner you should do another test. If you followed up with a long-term test and the result is 4 pCi/L or higher (0.02 WL or higher), take steps to fix your home (see page 175). If you followed up with a short-term test: The higher your short-term results, the more certain you can be that your home requires fixing. Consider taking steps to fix your home if the average result of your first and second tests is 4 pCi/L or higher (0.02 WL or higher).

•If your test result from either a long- or short-term test is below 4 pCi/L (below 0.02 WL), you may want to re-test your home in the future. Even radon levels below 4 pCi/L (0.02 WL) may pose some risk and should be lowered, according to the EPA.

remove radon from below the floor and foundation before it enters your home.

Depending on the amount of work involved, the extent of the radon problem, and the design of your home, you may choose to do the work yourself or to hire a radon contractor.

CHILDPROOFING YOUR HOME

M ost of us think of our home as a safe sanctuary from the outside world. Yet every home has its potential hazards, particularly for children. By identifying these hazards and learning how to prevent them, you can help ensure a safe home for your entire family.

ROOM-BY-ROOM REVIEW

Some rooms, such as the basement, garage, and kitchen, pose more hazards than others. For additional tips on keeping your child safe in these locations, see page 191.

Burn Prevention

•Turn handles in on cookware when using the stove.

•Limit range-top cooking to the back burners.

•Use an oven lock to prevent a hot oven from being opened.

•Check bath water temperature with temperature indictors.

Electricity

•Put safety covers on all electrical outlets. A variety of types are available. Look for ones that are self-closing.

•Use extension cords that have covers over their outlets. Always keep extension cords out of the reach of children.

•Unplug appliances when they're not in use.

•Know where the fuse box, circuit breaker, and outside switch box are located. Learn how to operate them.

Furnishings and Paint

•Anchor to the wall tall pieces of furniture, such as bookcases and chests.

•Place sharp-edged furniture, such as tables, out of the way of regular traffic. *AVOID* glass tabletops. Cover corners with protective cushions.

•Remove window blind cords or tie them up well out of reach, to prevent strangulation.

•Store knick-knacks and other objects well out of reach of children.

•Keep the liquor cabinet locked.

•Put childproof latches on all drawers, cupboards, cabinets and other areas containing unsafe items.

•Remove peeling or chipping paint from areas within your child's reach (see also Lead, page 189).

Doors, Windows, and Floors

•If you have sliding glass doors, place colorful stickers at your child's eye level. Be sure the floor in front of the doors is carpeted or covered with a rubber mat.

•Skidproof other areas of your house as well. Place padding under all area or smaller rugs.

•Keep chairs and other furniture away from all windows of your home.

•Use window guards on second story or higher windows to prevent falls.

•Install door locks or knob covers to prevent children from opening doors.

Stairs

•Use hardware-mounted safety gates at stairwells if you have an infant or small child. (Although it's tempting for you and older members of the family, avoid climbing over safety gates—your child may try to follow suit.)

•Cover stairs with carpet or rubber mats and check that the stair's handrail is steady and well secured.

•*DO NOT* allow your child to play near or on the stairs. Keep the area well lit and free of toys and other objects.

Small, Sharp, or Poisonous Objects

•Store safety pins, straight pins, needles, scissors, buttons, or other sharp and small objects well away from your child (see below for safety tips on toys). Keep small, round foods, such as grapes, nuts, and popcorn, out of reach too.

•For guidelines on protecting your child against poisonous substances, see Preventing Poisonings, page 186.

•Use a choke test tube (available at baby-supply stores) to test for small parts hazards.

Toys

•Large toys are best, particularly for a young child, since these toys are less likely to become stuck in a child's airway.

•Before buying, check each toy for small removable parts, sharp edges, or torn pieces.

•Read the toy's label—it contains important information about age suitability. If you are buying an electric toy, be sure it has UL (Underwriters Laboratories) approval.

•Give your child only crayons, paints, and markers that are nontoxic.

•Keep uninflated balloons or balloon pieces away from your child, and supervise your child when he plays with inflated balloons.

•If a toy contains batteries, make sure the batteries are not accessible to a child under age 5 years.

DON'T FOOL WITH FIREARMS

If you have a gun in your home, consider removing it—it's the safest thing you can do for your family. Wherever firearms are located, follow these safety procedures:

•Keep guns unloaded in a safe, locked area well out of the reach of children.

•Ensure that trigger locks and other safety features are used.

•Store ammunition separately from guns, also in a safe, well-locked area out of the reach of children.

•Keep older children's toys separate from those of younger children. For instance, chemistry sets, a popular choice among older children, are dangerous for younger ones.

•Be sure any toy box with a lid has safe hinges that will not pinch your child or close unexpectedly or has a fully removable lid. The box should also have holes to prevent suffocation, in case your child becomes trapped.

•*DO NOT* buy your child a toy gun. Some toy guns, particularly pellet and BB guns, can be unsafe. Moreover, if your child plays with toy guns, he may more easily mistake a real firearm for a toy gun.

•*DO NOT* buy toys that shoot small objects.

•*DO NOT* hang toys on long strings across an infant's crib or playpen. And *DO NOT* put his pacifier on a string or cord.

CHILDPROOFING CHECKLIST

BURN PREVENTION
•Turn handles in on cookware while on stove
•Use back burners on stove
•Use an oven lock
•Adjust hot-water heater to keep temperatures from reaching high levels
•Always check bath temperature

ELECTRICITY
•Put safety covers on all outlets
•Use extension cords with covers over outlets
•Unplug appliances not in use
•Locate and learn to use fuse box, circuit breaker, and switch box

FURNISHINGS AND PAINTS
•Anchor all tall furniture to wall
•Place sharp-edged furniture out of the way and cover corners with protective cushions
•Store knickknacks out of reach
•Lock liquor cabinet
•Put childproof latches on all drawers, cupboards, and cabinets
•Remove peeling or chipped paint
•Check wall paint for lead (see page 189)

WINDOWS, DOORS, AND FLOORS
•Remove or tie up window covering cords to prevent entanglement or strangulation
•Remove furniture near windows to stop children from reaching and opening windows
•Install locks on all windows
•Insert window guards on second-story or higher windows
•Place stickers on glass doors
•Install chain locks or knob covers on doors to prevent children from opening them
•Skid-proof all slippery areas with carpet or rubber mats

STAIRS
•Install safety gates
•Cover stairs with carpet or rubber mats
•Check handrails for stability
•Ensure your child doesn't play on or near stairs

(continued)

CHILDPROOFING CHECKLIST *(continued)*

SMALL, SHARP, OR POISONOUS OBJECTS
- Safely store in childproof cabinets
- Properly store poisonous materials (see page 186)

TOYS
- Choose suitable toys for child's age
- Check toys for small removable parts, sharp edges, or torn pieces
- Provide only nontoxic crayons, paints, and markers
- Discard uninflated balloons or balloon pieces
- Keep any toy batteries inaccessible to children under 5 years of age

- Separate older children's toys from those of younger children
- Choose a toy box with a lightweight lid, a hinge that stops the lid from slamming down, and holes in the side or front to allow air inside
- *DO NOT* hang toys on long strings across a crib or playpen
- *DO NOT* put a pacifier on a string or cord

GUN SAFETY
- Keep guns unloaded in a safe, locked area
- Store ammunition separately from guns
- Ensure that all gun safety features are used

SAFETY FOR THE ELDERLY

Elderly people are at greater risk for injuries in the home, so ensuring a safe environment should be a priority. Many of the points included in Childproofing (pages 176 to 180), Room-by-Room Safety (pages 191 to 194), and Safety Around the House and in the Garden (pages 195 to 198) are applicable, but there are additional measures you can take to safeguard a home for your elderly loved ones:

Fall Prevention
- Keep space open and free of clutter and poorly placed furniture
- Clean spills quickly
- Ensure adequate lighting in all rooms of the house (install night lights to permit a visible route to the bathroom at night)
- Make sure they wear non-slip, supportive shoes, and suitable clothing that fits
- Make sure they wear appropriate eyewear and use walking aids properly

•Obtain a personal or medical emergency response system (an electronic device that enables an elderly person to summon help in case of an emergency). These devices can be purchased, rented, or leased through national manufacturers, local distributors, hospitals, or social service agencies.

•Install a rail beside the toilet and bathtub. Place a mat and/or seat in the bathtub.

•Place an easy-to-reach light by the bedside.

Medications and Medical History

•Make a list of medications and doses and tape it to a convenient place (a kitchen cabinet, for instance). EMS personnel are usually trained to look there.

•Consider asking your doctor to make a copy of their baseline ECG (a record of the heart's electrical activity). On the back of it, include their past medical history, medications, and the doctor's contact numbers to carry in their wallet or purse.

ADDITIONAL GUIDELINES FOR HOMES WITH SENIORS

•Provide easy access to heating and cooling controls and the telephone.

•List all emergency numbers in large print.

•Keep all resuscitation or health care proxy documents in a convenient place.

•Ask your doctor how to access support services such as meals-on-wheels and home health aids, available in most communities.

FIREPROOFING YOUR HOME

When fires strike, common reactions are panic, anxiety, and confusion. That's why it's vital to be prepared for a fire in your home, not only with smoke alarms and firefighting equipment, but also with a family fire escape plan. By being prepared, you will safely confront and escape fires in your home.

FOR MORE INFORMATION...

Many organizations offer fire prevention advice; see page 249.

Install Smoke Alarms

Smoke alarms are a necessity in every home. Here's what you should know about them:

•Install smoke alarms on each level of your home and within 6 feet of all sleeping areas. If a member of your family sleeps with his door closed, install an alarm inside the room. Smoke alarms can be placed in two spots—on the ceiling, 4 inches from the nearest wall; or high on the wall, 4 to 12 inches from the ceiling. *DO NOT* place smoke alarms near a door, window, or fireplace.

•Keep your smoke alarms clean and dust-free with a vacuum or soft cloth.

•Test your smoke alarm at least once a month by pressing the test button and listening for the alarm. If necessary, replace the batteries. Check the smoke alarm batteries twice a year, when you change the clocks. New batteries should be installed at least once a year as a matter of course.

•Buy new smoke alarms every 10 years.

Furnish Your Home With Fire Extinguishers

Every home should be equipped with at least one fire extinguisher. Most home models contain dry chemicals that will be expelled in 8 to 25 seconds. There are four different ratings for fire extinguishers—A, B, C, and D (see Fire Extinguisher Types).

CARING FOR AND USING YOUR FIRE EXTINGUISHERS

•Most home fire extinguishers are designed for one-time use. This means that once you use the fire extinguisher, you must discard it and then buy a replacement.

•Store your fire extinguishers in easily accessible places away from heat sources and out of reach of your child.

•Learn how to operate your fire extinguishers *before* you need to use them. Teach other family members, except young children, how to use them as well. Extinguishers come with clear instructions that you

---

FIRE EXTINGUISHER TYPES

•A—for wood, paper cloth, upholstery, rubber, and other ordinary materials that burn easily
•B—for flammable liquids, such as paint, solvents, and oil
•C—for electrical equipment, wiring, fuse boxes, and appliances
•D—for metals

Your best bet is to buy multiple-rated ABC fire extinguishers that can be used for all types of fires.

should read carefully. Better yet, get training from your local fire department.

•Regularly check your fire extinguishers to confirm they are properly charged. A gauge or test button will indicate the pressure. If it's too low, follow the manufacturer's instructions on recharging or replacing the extinguisher. If you notice any damage, replace the extinguisher right away.

•Always consider your own safety when using a fire extinguisher. If you use the extinguisher and the fire doesn't immediately go out, drop it, leave the house, and call for help from a neighbor's house, cell phone (if you have one and it's handy), or nearby pay phone.

Develop a Family Fire Escape Plan For Your Home

•Draw a simple floor plan of your home. For each room, devise two escape plans, in case one is blocked by fire or smoke. Make sure everyone in your family understands and is familiar with the escape plans. Review them regularly.

•Store escape ladders by all bedroom windows on aboveground floors. Ensure that everyone knows how to use them.

•All security bars and locks on windows should be easy to open from the inside. If a key is needed, keep one near the window.

•Keep all exits from your home uncluttered and make sure they're well lit.

•Choose a safe place for your family to meet after escaping a fire.

•Conduct a fire drill at least twice a year. Instruct everyone to leave by one of the escape plans. (At the next drill, follow the second escape plan.) Practice escaping by crawling low. Some of the poisonous gases from fires will sink to the floor; others will rise to the ceiling. By crawling with your head about 1 or 2 feet above ground, you will be breathing the best air, at least temporarily.

•Teach your family to feel a closed door before opening it. If it feels hot, don't open the door. Use

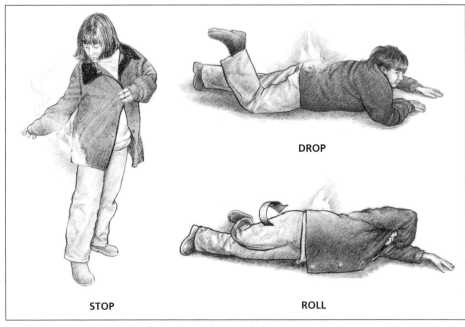

The stop, drop, and roll technique for putting out burning clothes.

a different exit or stay put and wait for help. Never crawl under the bed or hide in a closet—it will be difficult for emergency personnel to find you.

•Teach your child the "Stop, Drop, and Roll" technique for putting out burning clothes. This technique means stopping what you are doing, dropping to the ground, and covering your face and rolling back and forth until the flames go out.

Other Fireproofing Tips

•Keep matches and lighters in a safe, locked place well out of your child's reach.

•Never leave lit candles or fireplaces unattended.

•Be sure to place a fire screen directly in front of the fireplace.

•Use large, nonflammable ashtrays and empty them often if people smoke in your house. Always soak cigar or cigarette butts in water before throwing them out. *DO NOT* smoke in bed.

•Teach your child that grease fires in the kitchen should be put out with a lid, not with water.

BE SAFE WITH SPACE HEATERS

Like any electrical appliance, space heaters should be chosen and used with care, especially around children. The Good Housekeeping Institute has this advice:

HOW TO CHOOSE
•Choose only heaters tested at an independent lab such as UL or ETL.
•Make sure your model has tip-over protection (this feature should be listed on the box). The safest heaters turn themselves off if they're knocked over.
•Look for a model with a child-safety button to prevent your kids from turning the heat on or up. And teach them to stay at least 3 feet away from space heaters, no matter what.

HOW TO USE
•Choose a safe place for your space heater. Never set it in a high-traffic area.

Mount bathroom heaters on the wall, following only the manufacturer's directions. And never leave the house with a space heater running.
•Don't use an extension cord—most aren't designed to handle this much current.
•Never dry clothes over a space heater. They can be scorched or even catch on fire before the heat cuts off.
•Look for signs, such as a dented case, bent grill, or split or frayed wires at either end of the cord, that indicate your space heater needs replacing.
•Space heaters have been recalled in recent years for safety concerns. To get more details on recalls or to check on older models, contact the Consumer Product Safety Commission at 800-638-2772 or www.cpsc.gov.

•Keep your fireplace, furnace, chimney, space heaters, stove, other heat-producing appliances, and your home's electrical wiring well maintained and serviced.

•Only buy electric blankets that have been tested by an independent laboratory.

•Use space heaters safely (see Be Safe with Space Heaters, above).

•Keep clothing, blankets, furniture, and other flammable items well away from heat sources.

•Discard rags soaked with household cleaners.

•Consider installing a home fire sprinkler system.

•*DO NOT* overload outlets and extension cords.

HOLIDAYS AND CELEBRATIONS
•Keep party decorations, including Christmas trees, away from heat sources.

•Buy or rent flame-resistant or flame-retardant costumes.

•Use only outdoor lights that have been designed for that purpose.

•*AVOID* using candles as decorations. Try flashlights or torch lights instead.

•*DO NOT* leave cooking food unattended.

PREVENTING POISONINGS

Many substances that are found in the home can result in poisoning, including medications, vitamins, cleaners, fertilizers, cosmetics, paint remover, and some shampoos. Accidental poisonings most often occur in the early evening when parents are distracted or tired. Keeping a close eye on your children is vital, but properly storing and using all household chemicals and medications is equally important.

Lead, found in large amounts in some drinking water, paint, dust, and outdoor soil, is a big threat facing children today. Lead poisoning has few symptoms, so all lead sources in your home should be identified and removed.

Finally, don't forget about food poisoning. It's more common than you think. Problems are usually caused by undercooked meat and poultry, contaminated shellfish, and improperly stored perishable foods. By storing, handling, and cooking food in a safe manner, you can help prevent food poisoning from striking you and your family.

Food Poisoning

SHOPPING

•Buy fish or seafood that is stored on ice and that looks and smells fresh.

•*DO NOT* buy food that is out of date or that will be shortly.

•*DO NOT* buy cans that are dented or swollen or jars that are cracked, broken, or leaking.

•*DO NOT* buy cracked eggs.

BE PREPARED FOR POISONINGS

•Post by your phone: telephone numbers for doctors, local emergency medical services (EMS), and the local poison control center.
•Keep syrup of ipecac in your home first aid kit. This substance will induce vomiting but should be used *only* on the advice of a doctor or poison control center.

FOR MORE INFORMATION...

Several organizations including the US Food and Drug Administration (FDA) offer information on Food Safety. See page 249.

PROPER FOOD STORAGE

•Regularly check that your refrigerator and freezer are set at the right temperature—40°F or less for the refrigerator and 0°F for the freezer. *DO NOT* overfill these appliances; clean them often, discarding old and expired items.

•Freeze meat, fish, and poultry immediately, unless you plan to eat it within 2 days. If that's the case, carefully wrap the food in plastic and then place it in the refrigerator.

•Store eggs in their original containers in the body of the refrigerator. Egg holders on the door of a refrigerator tend to be warmer than other parts of the refrigerator and are not a good place to store your eggs.

•All cooked leftovers should be promptly refrigerated, within 2 hours of cooking. Separate leftovers into small portions in shallow containers so they cool quickly and evenly. *DO NOT* keep leftovers longer than 3 to 5 days.

•Keep all packed lunches as cool as possible, ideally in a refrigerator.

•Perishable picnic food should be chilled well in advance and then packed in a cooler.

PROPER FOOD HANDLING

•Wash your hands with soap and water, and clean your fingernails before handling food.

•Use two cutting boards (one for cutting vegetables and hot cooked meat; the other for raw meat, fish, and poultry). This will help keep bacteria in uncooked food away from raw or prepared foods.

•Wash all cutting boards, counters, and utensils with hot, soapy water. Using bleach or vinegar on these surfaces on a regular basis will help keep bacteria counts lower. Dish towels, cloths, and sponges can also harbor bacteria, so replace and/or wash them often.

•Keep foods at safe temperatures—32°F to 40°F for cold foods and over 140°F for hot foods.

•Wash all fruits and vegetables before eating or cooking. Wash cans and jars before opening them.

•Always defrost food in the refrigerator or microwave. *DO NOT* leave it sitting on the counter.

COOKING FOOD PROPERLY

•Marinate meat and other foods inside the refrigerator.

•Cook all meat and poultry thoroughly. Poultry and ground meat should never be pink in the middle. Using a meat/poultry thermometer is the best way to check. Most meat and poultry should be cooked to temperatures of 160°F or higher.

•When you stuff poultry, insert the cooled stuffing just before roasting. Better yet, cook the stuffing separately and then serve it alongside the poultry.

•Always cook eggs well, until the yolk and white are firm and not runny. Hard-boiled, firm fried, and scrambled eggs are the best choices. Sunnyside up, poached, and soft-boiled eggs are not recommended.

•Reheat foods thoroughly. If you see steam rising from the food, it has probably been heated sufficiently.

•If you can foods at home, be sure to follow canning instructions (from a reliable cookbook or other source) carefully.

•If you're barbecuing:

  •Always clean the grill first by heating it, and remove any food debris.

  •Pre-cook raw poultry, ribs, and other meats by microwaving or boiling. This will help ensure that the inside is cooked thoroughly.

  •Always use one plate to bring the food to the barbecue and another clean plate to take it away.

•If you're using the microwave:

  •Cover the food loosely with wax paper or heat-safe plastic wrap—this will create steam to help heat the food. Follow the instructions that came with your microwave regarding proper cooking containers and microwave times.

  •Rotate the food periodically to ensure even heating.

Household Chemicals and Other Products

GENERAL GUIDELINES

•Household and garden chemicals and cleaners are best stored in a basement or garage.

•Never store household products with food.

•If you're using a household product, be sure to finish the job and put it back in its proper storage place. Any interruptions or distractions can lead to potential poisonings. If you must stop what you're doing, take the product with you.

ADDITIONAL GUIDELINES FOR HOMES WITH CHILDREN

•Keep household and garden chemicals and cleaners in locked cupboards or on a high shelf.

•Always store household products in their original containers. If you store them in old juice or soda bottles, your child may confuse the poison for something to drink. Also, if your child does swallow a poison, you or someone else need to be able to identify it so that the correct treatment can be given.

•Products normally kept in your kitchen, such as dishwasher soap, should be stored in a cupboard with a safety latch. Remember to keep the cupboard closed at all times.

•Buy childproof containers when possible.

•Even shampoo, cream, perfume, and other hair and body products can be poisonous. Be diligent about storing them out of reach as well.

Lead *GOOD HOUSEKEEPING INSTITUTE REPORT*

•Test the paint, water, and soil in and around your home for lead levels. If high readings are found, take steps to remove the lead sources. It's best to leave this up to an experienced professional. For more information about lead and what to do about it, call 800-424-LEAD.

DID YOU KNOW...

Mixing chlorine and ammonia can produce life-threatening toxic fumes. Always check the labels of your cleaning agents carefully.

•*DO NOT* store anything in ceramicware, especially acidic liquids such as orange juice, wine, or vinegar. Refilling a flea-market mug or old china all day long with hot, acidic beverages is also a bad idea, especially if you're pregnant (lead will be passed on to your unborn child).

•If your home has any lead pipes, or solder in the plumbing, let the water run until it's as cold as it's going to get (especially in the morning) before drinking or cooking with it. Lead concentrations are highest in water left standing in pipes for long periods of time.

•*DO NOT* let your child play with or put in his mouth other sources of lead, such as colored newsprint, old utensils with painted handles, or old painted toys.

•If you suspect that your child may have been exposed to high lead levels, take him to the doctor to have his blood lead levels checked and to receive treatment.

•Discuss lead poisoning prevention with your doctor.

Medications

Medications—prescription, over-the-counter, even vitamins—are the most common cause of childhood poisonings. Responsible use and storage of medication in your home is vital for all family members, young and old.

GENERAL GUIDELINES

•Always read medication labels carefully, and only give the recommended dose. Never give one person's prescription medication to someone else.

•Go through your medicine cabinet on a regular basis. Flush old or expired medication down the toilet or drain. Then rinse the container with water and discard it.

ADDITIONAL GUIDELINES FOR HOMES WITH CHILDREN

•Keep all medications in a locked cabinet well out of your child's reach.

•Buy medication in childproof containers when you can, but don't let these containers lull you into a false sense of security. Childproof containers are not 100% effective.

•Learn about important differences between infant- and toddler-strength acetaminophen. Ask your doctor or pharmacist to explain the differences and help you choose the right product and strength for your child. Remember, never give a child aspirin. Its use may cause Reye's syndrome, a disease that affects the body's organs, particularly the brain and liver.

Plants and Flowers

Both plants and flowers in and around your home can be dangerous if your child eats or puts them in his mouth.

•Always identify which plants and flowers are poisonous. This information is available in plant and flower books or at your local nursery.

•Teach your children to keep all plants and flowers out of their mouths.

•*AVOID* planting poisonous flowers and plants in your garden, or placing them in your home. Check with a gardening resource or poison control center if you have specific concerns.

ROOM-BY-ROOM SAFETY

Although accidents can happen anywhere in your home, some rooms, such as the basement, bathroom, garage, and kitchen, are more hazardous than others. By paying special attention to these areas, you can help ensure that safety is a common theme throughout your home.

Basement/Storage/Laundry Rooms

GENERAL GUIDELINES

•Be sure your furnace, vents, flues, and other heating/cooling system components are regularly maintained and serviced.

DID YOU KNOW...

Childproof containers are not 100% effective. Keep all medications out of the reach of children.

CHILDPROOFING YOUR HOME

Remember, special precautions are needed throughout your home if you have children. See also Childproofing Your Home (details on page 176) and Preventing Poisonings (details on page 186).

•Keep your entire basement clean, dustfree, and well lit.

•If you store firewood in your basement, place it in a separate room, well away from heat sources.

•Make sure washer and dryer doors are always closed. Unplug the iron and put it away right after you're finished using it.

•Regularly clean the lint screen in your clothes dryer. *DO NOT* run your dryer when you aren't at home or when you're sleeping.

•*DO NOT* keep rags soaked in household chemicals. Discard them immediately.

ADDITIONAL GUIDELINES FOR HOMES WITH CHILDREN

•Supervise young children when they are in the basement until they are older and more responsible. Use a simple latch placed high on the door to prevent your child's entry into the basement (particularly a storage/unfinished basement).

•All paints, varnishes, thinners, laundry products, and other household chemicals should be kept in their original containers and stored safely in a locked cupboard or high on a shelf, out of reach and out of sight of children. (For more information, see Household Chemicals and Other Products, page 189.)

•Store all nails, screws, hammers, and other tools safely out of your child's reach.

•Lock all freezers and additional refrigerators.

Bathroom

GENERAL GUIDELINES

•To prevent hot water burns, set the thermostat on your home water heater to lower than 110°F.

•Keep all electrical appliances, such as hair dryers or curlers, away from water. When these items are plugged in, never leave them unattended. When not in use, unplug and put them away.

•Place a rubber mat or nonskid decals in the bathtub and shower. Install safety railings in your bath and shower and around your toilet if you have an elderly or disabled person in your home.

ADDITIONAL GUIDELINES FOR HOMES WITH CHILDREN

•Always test the water temperature before allowing your child to bathe or shower. Use your forearm to test the water, keeping it immersed for several seconds.

•Always supervise young children when they take a bath or shower.

•Store all medications in a locked cabinet out of reach and sight of children. A cool, dry place is the best environment for most medications. (For more information, see Medications, page 190.)

•Place razors, perfumes, hairdryers, and cosmetics in a drawer or cupboard with a safety latch.

•Store shampoo, soap, and toothpaste out of reach of young children.

•Always keep the bathroom door closed and the toilet seat down.

•*DO NOT* keep bathroom cleaning products under the sink. Keep them in your basement in a locked cupboard or high on a shelf.

Garage

GENERAL GUIDELINES

•Keep all pesticides, fertilizers, and other chemicals in their original containers.

•*DO NOT* run your car in a closed garage.

ADDITIONAL GUIDELINES FOR HOMES WITH CHILDREN

•Supervise young children when they are in a garage until they are older and more responsible.

•Always keep car doors locked.

•Store containers of pesticides, fertilizers, and other chemicals in a locked cabinet or high on a shelf. (For more information, see Household Chemicals and Other Products, page 189.)

•Store all garden and power tools, as well as other

equipment such as ladders, cords, and ropes well out of reach of children.

•*DO NOT* let your child play with the automatic garage door opener if you have one.

Kitchen

GENERAL GUIDELINES

•Post all telephone numbers for doctors, local emergency medical services (EMS), the local poison control center, and police and fire departments near the phone.

•Unplug appliances, such as the toaster, microwave, and food processor, when not in use and when you are trying to remove a stuck object, such as bread in the toaster.

•Prevent falls by cleaning up all spills right away.

•If you have an area rug in the kitchen, it should be rubber-backed.

•*DO NOT* leave cooking food, particularly oil or other flammable products, unattended.

ADDITIONAL GUIDELINES FOR HOMES WITH CHILDREN

•Store dishwasher soap and items you use daily in a cupboard with safety latches. All household chemicals should be stored in a locked cabinet or high on a shelf—in your basement if possible. (For more information, see Household Chemicals and Other Products, page 189.)

•Use safety latches on all drawers and cupboards containing sharp utensils, cookware, and other heavy items.

•Keep all appliances, such as the toaster, microwave, or food processor, away from the countertop edge.

•Cook on back burners whenever possible and turn pot handles toward the back of the stove.

•Keep your child's high chair away from busy or dangerous areas such as the stove, countertop, sink, and phone.

DID YOU KNOW...

Many home fires start in the kitchen. See Fireproofing Your Home, page 181, for more fire prevention details.

SAFETY AROUND THE HOUSE AND IN THE GARDEN

S afety at home doesn't apply just indoors but also to the garden, backyard, and house exterior. Barbecues, pools, swings, and slides are just some of the things around your home that require careful accident prevention.

Exterior of Your House

•Regularly clean your eaves and gutters. Your roof and chimney should be well maintained.

•When using a ladder, have someone stabilize it from below and remain there until you descend. Keep your child well away from the ladder.

•Ensure that all steps and railings are in good condition.

•In winter, shovel snow daily to keep the entrances to your home clear and safe. Sprinkle salt or other anti-icing substances on steps and sidewalks to prevent icy conditions and falls.

•*DO NOT* allow any member of your family to go on the roof. Only trained roofing company employees should venture there.

Barbecues

FOR ALL TYPES OF BARBECUES

•Position your barbecue far from anything that will burn, such as your home, garage, or garden.

•Keep a container of water nearby to douse any flames.

•When you're using the barbecue, keep children and pets well away.

•Always use proper barbecuing utensils and wear an apron and oven mitts.

•*DO NOT* leave a lit barbecue unattended.

•*DO NOT* use a barbecue inside the house.

•*AVOID* adding oil or grease to the food you're barbecuing.

IF YOU HAVE A CHARCOAL BARBECUE

•Use a small amount of starter fluid (never gasoline) to start the fire. *DO NOT* add more fluid if the fire is weak or dying—try adding more charcoal instead. Keep an eye on the charcoal as it becomes hot.

•Once you've finished barbecuing, soak the charcoal with water and then discard it.

•*DO NOT* attempt to move the barbecue until it is well cooled.

IF YOU HAVE A GAS BARBECUE

•Always store the gas cylinder outside and use caution when you have it refilled.

•To guarantee that your tank has been filled correctly, check out one of the cylinder-exchange programs at supermarkets, mass merchandisers, home centers, convenience stores, and gas stations. For around $15, you can exchange your empty tank for one that's been inspected and prefilled by a certified technician. These new tanks will have leakproof valves.

•Always transport the tank in an upright position.

•Each time you reconnect the cylinder, check for leaks by brushing soapy water over the connections. If bubbles form, you need to tighten the connections.

•When the barbecue is not in use, ensure that the gas valve is turned off.

•Always follow the manufacturer's instructions for using and maintaining the barbecue.

•If the barbecue valve or cylinder is damaged, stop using it immediately and have a trained service technician repair or replace it.

Garden

•Regularly trim trees and bushes that hang too close to your home or power lines. If the job is a big one, hire a professional.

•When using garden tools, such as lawnmowers or chain saws, wear sturdy shoes or boots, long pants, and safety glasses. Clear the area of rocks, sticks, or other objects that may be thrown by the lawnmower. *DO NOT* use a lawnmower around children or pets.

•Carefully store all garden tools in a securely locked shed or garage.

•When using pesticides, be sure to follow directions carefully and pay attention to the stated safety precautions, such as wearing rubber gloves, and staying off grass for a specified period of time. Always keep pesticides and other garden chemicals in a locked cabinet well out of reach of children and pets.

•*AVOID* planting poisonous flowers and plants in your garden. Check with a gardening resource or poison control center if you have specific concerns.

Pool

Pool safety must be strictly followed to protect everyone who uses it

•Place a regulation fence around the entire pool area and keep the gates locked when the pool is not in use.

•Always remove the pool cover before swimming.

•Keep a life preserver or another flotation device near the pool.

•Learn CPR (see page 12).

•Take a basic water safety course offered by first aid organizations (see page 257).

•Consider installing an alarm on the gate of the pool and a special pool alarm for the water. A pool alarm will tell you when anything heavy falls into the pool, or if there is a sound or change in pressure underwater.

•*DO NOT* let anyone swim alone, even adults. Children should be closely supervised by adults at all times.

•*DO NOT* allow running or other games around the pool.

•*DO NOT* allow diving into an above-ground pool or in any water less than 9 feet deep.

WATER AND BOATING SAFETY

Keeping safe around water also includes taking precautions at the beach or lake or while boating. For safety guidelines in these types of settings, see page 212.

•*DO NOT* take drugs or alcohol just before or while swimming.

EXERCISE CARE WITH POOL CHEMICALS

•Safely store all pool chemicals outside your home, well away from heat sources and out of reach of children.

•Before buying chemicals, inspect the container for any damage. If a container becomes damaged later, dispose of the chemicals immediately.

•Carefully add chemicals according to the manufacturer's instructions. Be sure no one is in the pool when you do it.

Slides, Swings, and Sandboxes

•Be sure there is grass, sand, or another soft substance under the play equipment.

•Swings should be sling-style and constructed of canvas or hard rubber.

•Slides should be 6 feet high or less for children under 8 years of age. For older children, slides should be no taller than 8 feet.

•All play equipment should be regularly inspected and maintained. Cover any sharp edges or screws with plastic caps. If the equipment is old, unsteady, or corroded, consider replacing it.

•Regularly clean and dry out a sandbox. Cover it to keep out domestic and wild animals.

•Always supervise children on play equipment.

•Ensure that your child doesn't wear long dangling clothing that could become caught in the play equipment.

•Teach your child not to place his tongue on play equipment or other metal objects, especially in winter. In summer, check any metal slides to make sure they aren't too hot to play on.

PLAYING IT SAFE WHEN YOU'RE AWAY FROM HOME

SAFETY PREPARATION BEFORE TRAVELING

You've picked your destination, booked your accommodations, and decided how you'll get there. But before leaving, you also need to consider your health when traveling.

The best way to stay healthy when you're away from home is to research your destination, know the local conditions, and be prepared for them. Here are some important but simple steps you should take before leaving on your trip.

What You Should Do

• Ensure that your health insurance covers you and your family en route and at your destination. If not, arrange for additional travel insurance.

• If necessary, get immunized. Talk to your family doctor at least 6 weeks in advance of your trip about the shots you will need.

• Research your destination, and find out how to get medical help while you're there. If you're traveling overseas, try to learn a few key words in the local language. If you have a special medical condition, carry a note that explains your condition in the local language and a medical ID bracelet or necklace.

• If you wear prescription eyeglasses, take an extra pair along. And don't forget to bring your sunglasses as well.

• Carry all your prescription medication with you. If you're traveling on a plane, take your medication on board with you. Pack more medications than you need, although always take it only as directed. Keep the medications in their original containers along with copies of the original prescriptions.

FOR MORE INFORMATION...

Before you travel, a good site to visit is the Centers for Disease Control and Prevention Web site, which offers a wealth of information for travelers; see page 257 for more information.

MOTION SICKNESS

Motion sickness occurs when the body is subjected to movement in different directions (for example, in a car or train) or in situations where it becomes hard to focus on the horizon (such as on a boat). Symptoms of motion sickness include fatigue, dizziness, and nausea. You can help prevent motion sickness by eating light before traveling and placing yourself in areas where movement is felt the least (such as the interior of a ship, the center of a bus, or near the wing of an airplane). Make sure to face forward and keep your eyes on distant non-moving objects if possible. Several over-the-counter medications, such as Dramamine (dimenhydrinate), are available that may prevent or decrease symptoms of motion sickness. For longer trips, talk to your doctor about prescription medications that may help combat this condition.

AIR TRAVEL

TRAVELING BY AIRPLANE INCLUDES ADDITIONAL MEDICAL PRECAUTIONS

•Take a walk through the plane cabin once every hour or so to prevent swollen legs or ankles and possible blood clots. If you're prone to swelling in these areas, wear support stockings.

•To relieve ear pain during takeoff and landing, swallow, yawn, or chew gum. If you have a cold with nasal congestion, ask your doctor about taking a deconges-tant before flying.

•To help prevent jet lag, drink lots of nonalcoholic fliuds during your flight. Also consider taking melatonin to pre-vent jet lag.

•If you have lung or heart disease, you may need supplemental oxygen during air travel. Ask your doctor and, if neces-sary, make arrangements with the airline well in advance of your trip.

•Consider how time zones and your travel itinerary may affect your medication schedule. Speak with your doctor about whether any adjustments are needed in your medication schedule.

•If you use injectable medications (insulin, for instance), take a note from your doctor explaining this fact to immigration officials, who may be concerned that you're carrying syringes and medication. Be sure to take your own syringes.

•In addition to your prescription medications, pack a small medicine kit, containing

•Acetaminophen, ibuprofen, or aspirin (remember that aspirin should be given only to adults).

•Antidiarrheal and antinausea medication

•Antihistamines and decongestants

•Antibacterial ointment

•Sunscreen (SPF 15 or higher)

•For some parts of the world, consider bringing water-purifying pills or a mechanical water purifier, a permethrin-impregnated bed net to keep out mosquitoes, and antimalaria pills (these pills must be started 2 weeks before your departure).

•If you have a particular medical condition, be sure to check with your doctor before traveling. And take a copy of your medical record with you.

AUTOMOBILE SAFETY

Safe Driving Tips

Today's cars are safer than yesterday's, with shatterproof windshields, air bags, shoulder and lap seat belts, and headrests. But these features are not the whole story. Your driving skills, including your response to other drivers and road conditions are just as important. Here are some tips to help you become a safer, more aware driver all year round.

•*DO NOT* drive if you're sleepy; if you have had alcohol, medication, or any illicit drugs that may interfere with your ability to drive; or if you feel deeply angry or upset.

•Have your eyes checked. If necessary, wear the appropriate prescription eyewear when you drive. If the conditions are sunny or bright, use sunglasses.

•Be sure your car insurance is up to date.

•Put on your seat belt. Have all passengers belt up as well. If an infant or child is in the car, place him in the appropriate safety seat (for details, see page 203). Be sure all children are suitably restrained in the back seat.

•Always follow the rules of the road, such as signaling before moving into traffic or changing lanes, obeying all traffic signs and lights, giving bicyclists plenty of room, driving within the speed limit, and keeping at least two car lengths between you and the car in front.

•Avoid aggressive drivers, and don't behave aggressively yourself.

•Consider taking a driving improvement course.

•If you're an elderly driver (or know someone who is), adopt an objective, reasoned approach to your driving skills.

Safety Features in Your Car

SEAT BELTS

There's no doubt about it, seat belts work. When used properly, they are the most effective way of

FOR MORE INFORMATION...

The American Automobile Association (AAA), the National Highway Traffic Safety Administration (NHTSA), and the National Safety Council all offer valuation information on auto safety, car seats, and more; see page 241 for details.

ITEMS TO KEEP IN YOUR CAR IN CASE OF AN EMERGENCY

There are several items you should keep in your car in case of emergencies.

YEAR-ROUND ITEMS
- Squeegee and brush for cleaning windshield
- Paper towels and cloths
- Windshield washer fluid
- Water in a plastic container for the radiator (to use if car overheats)
- Road maps and compass
- Booster cables
- Gas siphon
- Rope (at least 16 feet)
- Flashlight and extra batteries
- Warning light or road flares
- Tool kit—a jack and other tools for fixing a flat tire, screwdrivers of various sizes, and wirecutters
- Repair wire and duct tape
- Inflated, undamaged spare tire
- Heat warmers (to warm your hands)
- Waterproof matches
- Fire extinguisher (BC type—see page 182)
- Cellular phone (if you have one) or change for a pay phone.
- First aid kit. A kit for your car can be similar to your home first aid kit (see Home First Aid Kit, page 2), with the addition of disposable wipes. Remember that many medications, such as epinephrine, are affected by extremes of temperature. (When in doubt, check the label.) It is best not to store medications in your car, but to take them along with you on a long car trip or as needed.

IN WINTER CONDITIONS
- Ice scraper and brush
- Antifreeze windshield washer fluid
- Shovel
- Sand or salt
- Extra, warm clothing and footwear
- Emergency food pack and bottled drinking water (especially if severe conditions are anticipated)
- Blanket

preventing serious injury and death from car accidents. Seat belts should be used every time you or a family member is in the car (for children weighing less than 70 pounds, safety seats should be used—see page 203). Putting on your seat belt should become automatic, just like closing the car door. If your car doesn't have an automatic reminder signal to fasten seat belts, leave a note posted to your sun visor or dashboard.

Shoulder and lap belts offer the best protection. If your car only has lap belts, be sure to use them—they will help protect you in the event of an accident.

To do their job, seat belts must be properly secured to the car and correctly adjusted for the passenger in order to fit snugly without being uncomfortable. Shoulder belts should fit across your shoulder and upper thigh bones.

Pregnant women should take some care in positioning the seat belt—the shoulder part of the belt should be placed over the collarbone and the lap portion below, not over, the abdomen, low on the upper thighs.

CHILD SAFETY SEATS

Across the United States, by law all children must be restrained by a safety seat or properly adjusted seat belt. Although not legislated, there is a second rule you should always follow—*all* children, including infants, should ride in the back seat.

Infants and young children need safety seats because their bodies can't take the pressure of an ordinary seat belt when a car accident occurs. A safety seat is effective only when it is chosen, installed, and used properly. The NHTSA periodically updates their standards to ensure that safety seats are safe and easy to install (for details, see page 204).

Choosing a Safety Seat

•Choose a safety seat that is the right size and model for your child's age and weight and that fits into your car.

•A safety seat should meet all federal safety standards. It should also have a model number and a sticker with a manufacture date after January 1, 1981 (if made before then, the seat may not meet strict safety standards). To find out if your seat has been recalled, contact the US Consumer Products Safety Commission (page 238).

•It's best to purchase a safety seat that is no more than 10 years old, although some manufacturers state that seats should be used only for 6 years. Check the instruction booklet for your manufacturer's recommendations.

•*DO NOT* buy a seat that has been in an accident, has cracks in the frame, has missing parts, or does not come with the manufacturer's instruction booklet.

SAFETY SEAT STANDARDS

The NHTSA standards ensure that child safety seats are safe and easy to install. It is important to keep up to date on the changing developments in child safety seat laws in order to select the most appropriate safety seat for your child.

THE LOWER ANCHORS AND TETHERS FOR CHILDREN (LATCH) SYSTEM

As of September 1, 2002, federal law requires that nearly all passenger vehicles and child safety seats manufactured be equipped with the LATCH system. The system is designed to standardize and simplify the installation of child safety seats without using the vehicle's seat belt system.

TETHER STRAP AND ANCHOR

LATCH-equipped vehicles have two sets of small bars, or anchors, located in the back seat where the cushions meet and a top anchor. LATCH-equipped safety seats have a lower set of attachments that fasten to the vehicle's lower anchor. Most forward-facing child safety seats also have a top strap, or tether, that attaches to the top anchor in the vehicle. Together, the anchors, attachments, and tether make up the LATCH system.

If your vehicle isn't LATCH equipped, use the seat belt and, if available, a top tether when securing your safety seat. If your child safety seat isn't LATCH equipped, it's still safe if it has been correctly installed using a seat belt, has *not* been recalled, and has *not* been damaged.

SAFETY RATINGS

In June 2003, the NHTSA announced its initial set of ratings for child safety seats based on their ease of use. Under this rating system, child safety seats (including booster seats) are given overall grades of A, B, or C. These grades are also used to rate the following:
•Whether the seat is preassembled or requires assembly after purchase
•Clarity of labeling attached to the seat
•Clarity of written instructions on the seat's proper use
•Ease of securing a child in the seat
•Whether the seat has features that make it easier to install in a vehicle

To get updates on child safety seat information, call 888-327-4236 or go to www. nhtsa.dot.gov (see also page 242).

•Once you've bought the car seat, send in the registration card right away, so you can be notified of any recalls.

Using a Safety Seat

•Consult your vehicle owner's manual for fastening the seat securely in the car.

•Always use the car seat according to the manufacturer's instruction booklet.

•Regularly check your child's safety seat to ensure that it is in good working order. Repair any minor problems. *DO NOT* use a seat that is clearly damaged or that has been in an accident.

•An infant weighing 20 pounds or less and under 1 year of age should be placed in an infant-only or rear-facing convertible seat, both of which must be positioned facing the back of the car. (Never substitute a household infant play seat.) Harness straps must fit snugly over the infant's shoulders and between his legs. Place the harness retainer clip at mid-chest, armpit level.

•A child weighing 20 to 40 pounds and more than 1 year of age should be placed in a convertible forward-facing seat with a full harness. If the seat has a harness retainer clip, place it at your child's armpit level to hold the harness straps on his shoulders.

•A child weighing 40 to 80 pounds should be placed in a booster seat facing forward—see "Boost 'Em Before You Buckle 'Em." Never substitute a household booster seat for this purpose. There are three types of booster seats:

  •A belt-positioning booster (a booster without a shield) that must be used with both the car's lap belt and shoulder belt. Make sure the lap belt fits low and tight, and the shoulder belt stays on your child's shoulders and close to his chest.

  •Boosters with removable shields. Remove the shield to make sure lap and shoulder belts fit correctly. A booster with a shield may be used if your car has only lap belts, although this type of booster doesn't provide adequate protection for your child's upper body. Shield boosters *cannot* be used for children weighing more than 40 pounds, and children weighing less than 40 pounds may be ejected from a shield booster in a rollover crash. If your car has only lap belts, consider having shoulder harnesses installed so that you can use belt-positioning booster seats.

  •High-backed boosters, used as belt-positioning boosters. Most models have a clip or strap that holds the shoulder belt in place.

"BOOST 'EM BEFORE YOU BUCKLE 'EM"

The NHTSA says "boost 'em before you buckle 'em"—that is, use a booster seat when your child has outgrown his car seat. Children under 80 pounds and less than 4 feet, 9 inches, are too small to be safely restrained in the car's lap or lap/shoulder belt in the event of an accident; and a properly fitted booster seat will provide the extra protection they need.

•Your child should continue using the belt-positioning booster seat until his weight is more than 80 pounds and he is large enough so that the car's seat belt rests across his pelvis, not his abdomen, and he can sit with his back against the vehicle's car seat, knees bent over the seat edge with feet flat on the floor.

AIR BAGS

Starting in model year 1998, all passenger vehicles are required to have driver and passenger (dual) air bags. The same is true for all light trucks beginning in model year 1999. "Air Bag," "SRS" (supplemental restraint system), or "SIR" (supplemental inflatable restraint) indicate that air bags are present. If you're unsure whether your car has air bags, check your vehicle owner's manual.

Supplementing the protection provided by seat belts, air bags inflate at speeds up to 200 mph to cushion adults as they move forward in a front-end crash. Airbags have saved many lives and prevented many injuries. In a very few cases, people have been injured or killed by air bags, mostly because they have been improperly restrained or too close to the air bag when it started to deploy.

You can reduce air bag risk by

•Always placing an infant in a rear-facing infant seat in the back seat.

•Always placing children, aged 1 to 12, in the back seat and using the correct restraint (see page 203).

•Always buckling your own seat belt and keeping 10 inches between the center of the air bag and your breastbone.

Since January 1998, you have had the choice of having an on-off switch for air bags installed in your vehicle if you, or a user of your vehicle, is in one of the following risk groups:

•You *must* transport infants in a rear-facing infant seat in the front passenger seat (due to a special health need that requires monitoring, for instance).

•You *must* transport children, aged 1 to 12, in the front passenger seat.

•You *cannot* change your usual driving position to keep 10 inches between the center of the steering wheel (the center of the airbag) and the center of your breastbone.

•You have a medical condition and your doctor advises that the risk from the airbag deploying is greater than the risk of injury in a crash if the airbag is turned off.

If you, or a user of your vehicle, is eligible, you must fill out a NHTSA request form, available at state motor vehicle offices and at some auto dealers and repair shops. You can also call the NHTSA Hotline or visit its Web site (see page 242). If your request is approved, the NHTSA will send you a letter authorizing an auto dealer or repair shop to install an on-off switch in your vehicle.

RECREATIONAL SAFETY

Bicycling and In-Line Skating

Both bicycling and in-line skating are fun-filled activities for the whole family that can improve fitness, control weight, and strengthen and tone muscles. By using precautions and common sense, you can enjoy bicycling and in-line skating without serious injury.

BICYCLING

Preparation

•Always wear a helmet. Many states require that bicyclists wear helmets, particularly those under 18 years of age. Helmets save lives and will protect you and your family from serious head injury. Buy a helmet from a trained dealer who can fit it properly. The helmet should have a label from the Snell Memorial Foundation, ANSI (American National Standards Institute), ASTM (American Society for Testing and Materials), or the Consumer Product Safety Commission (see pages 238 and 242). Choose a helmet that fits snugly and

FOR MORE INFORMATION...

Organizations, such as the Bicycle Helmet Safety Institute and the International Inline Skating Association, offer safety and other information on bicycling and skating. See page 243.

comfortably. *DO NOT* buy a cracked helmet or one that doesn't fit properly.

•Choose the right clothing. You should be dressed in bright, close-fitting clothes that won't get caught in the bicycle parts. If necessary, wear leg bands or clips to keep pant legs away from the bike.

•Put all items in a backpack, or secure them to a fixed bike carrier. Your hands must be completely free to operate the bike.

•If you're going mountain (off-road) biking, consider carrying essential first aid supplies along with your bike repair kit.

When You Ride

•Obey all traffic rules and remember to use the correct hand signals.

•Avoid riding in heavy traffic. Be on the lookout for car doors opening unexpectedly or cars pulling out of driveways.

•Have a bell or other signal on your bike to warn others you're there.

•Children shouldn't cycle at dusk or in the dark. Adults riding at these times must do so with caution using bike reflectors (front and rear), a headlight, and a reflective vest. Always stick to well-lit areas.

•*DO NOT* allow your children to hang onto a moving vehicle while on a bike.

•*DO NOT* let another person ride on the handlebars or fender of your bike.

•*AVOID* riding in rainy conditions. Try to steer clear of potholes and slippery surfaces.

IN-LINE SKATING

•Always wear a helmet (see page 207), as well as wrist, elbow, and knee pads.

•Wear reflective, light-colored clothing, particularly if you skate at dusk or early in the morning.

•Children and adolescents should stick to dead-end streets or those that are blocked off.

•If you're new to in-line skating, practice first in an empty parking lot or outdoor arena before hitting the roads. Learn how to stop quickly and fall safely.

•Keep an eye out for road debris and defects, and avoid them whenever possible. Keep well clear of traffic.

Hiking and Camping

Enjoying the great outdoors is a favorite pastime for many Americans. Hiking and camping can be a fun, healthy way for your family to experience true adventure together. But remember to make safety a priority when you're planning and partaking in your nature outing.

Plan Ahead

•Plan your hiking and camping trip carefully. Choose a hiking trail that is suitable to your fitness level and the age and stamina of your child. Consider all the supplies you will need while you're outdoors. Find out as much as you can about where you're going, including any possible hazards or obstacles.

•Relay your plan to a responsible friend or relative. Tell him when you'll be leaving and returning. Always stick to your initial plan. If it changes, be sure to inform the person immediately.

•Plan to go with other people. Camping or hiking alone is not a good idea, particularly if an emergency situation arises—you'll need more than one set of hands.

•Learn how to use a map and compass. Teach older children to use them as well.

•Identify where help can be found, such as the nearest pay phone or ranger station. You can usually obtain this information when you check into a park or camping area.

•Take along a well-stocked first aid kit on your camping trip. While hiking, carry it with you in a backpack. In addition to a first aid kit, you will need some other essential supplies (see Essential Camping Supplies, page 210).

•Go through the A to Z First Aid section (pages

FOR MORE INFORMATION…

There are several Web sites devoted to hiking and camping. See page 244 for details.

ESSENTIAL CAMPING SUPPLIES

•A good supply of your prescription medication (if applicable) and a first-aid kit (see Home First Aid Kit, page 2)
•Sewing needles (to remove splinters)
•An extra pair of eyeglasses (if you wear eyeglasses)
•Sunglasses and sunscreen
•Insect repellent
•Water-purifying tablets or device
•Pocket knife

•Waterproof matches and candles
•Space blanket (compact metal blanket)
•Flares and a whistle
•Flashlight with extra batteries
•Communication equipment such as a cellular phone, VHF radio, geographic (GPS) locator, or walkie-talkies
•Compass and map
•Plenty of drinking water

27 to 172). Pay special attention to Broken Bones, Frostbite, Hypothermia, Snake Bites, Sprains and Strains, and Tick Bites. Be sure to take this book along with you for easy reference.

•Plan each meal you will have on your trip, keeping in mind that you will have limited cooking resources. Always pack more food than you think you'll need. Be sure to pack the food well, so it is sealed and waterproof.

•Before you leave, check the weather report. If the outlook is poor, it may be wise to consider postponing your trip until better weather arrives.

What To Wear

•Pack plenty of warm clothes and dress in layers so that they can be removed if you get too hot.

•Cover as much skin as you can to help prevent tick and other insect bites, scrapes, and exposure to poisonous or irritating plants.

•Be sure to take along hats and rain gear. If the weather is cold, pack warm mittens or gloves and scarves.

•Wear proper hiking boots that fit well and are well broken in. Be sure to wear thick socks for good foot protection.

Camping Tips

•Pitch your tent in a clean, dry area on level ground. Consider where water will run if it rains.

•Always keep tents zipped closed to keep insects out. With a flashlight, check your tent for insects and other small creatures before you go to bed.

•Build your campfire on bare ground, stone, or other firesafe areas. Be sure the fire is far away from flammable items such as your tent, trees, or dry grass. Keep a close eye on your children around a campfire and ensure it is completely extinguished before you leave or go to bed.

Hiking Tips

•Try to stay away from tall grass and dense woods to avoid ticks and other creatures that bite.

•Drink plenty of water to prevent dehydration. Stop for regular snacks and meals.

•Remind your child to stay away from all plants and wild berries.

HOW TO PREVENT ALTITUDE SICKNESS (MOUNTAIN SICKNESS)

If you're hiking in the mountains, prepare yourself for reduced levels of oxygen that occur at higher altitudes. In some people, reduced oxygen levels can lead to altitude sickness. It's impossible to predict who will suffer from this condition. Fortunately, there are steps you can take to help prevent or reduce the symptoms of altitude sickness.

•Start your climb at a level below 9,000 feet. Rest at that altitude for a day, so your body can get used to (acclimatize to) the conditions.

•Climb slowly—no more than 3,000 feet per day. Stop and rest whenever you feel tired or out of breath.

•Always sleep at lower altitudes at night. If you're above 11,000 feet during the day, descend to 9,000 feet or lower to sleep.

•Ask your doctor about the prescription medications acetazolamide (Diamox) and dexamethasone (Decadron) that can prevent or lessen the symptoms of altitude sickness.

•*DO NOT* drink alcohol or smoke cigarettes.

For the signs and symptoms of altitude sickness and ways to treat it, see page 33.

•If you're hiking in winter, keep an eye out for the signs and symptoms of frostbite (see page 102) or hypothermia (see page 117).

•Be sure to leave enough daylight to set up camp or to return to your campsite.

•To avoid bear and other animal attacks, pay attention to warnings posted. Find out about local animal habitats, food sources, and signs. A park official can be a good guide on whether there are any animals to avoid, including bears, in the area—and how to steer clear of them.

•*AVOID* walking too close to cliff edges, loose rocks, or slippery surfaces.

Water and Boating Safety

The lure of water is strong for many people, particularly when the weather is warm and balmy. What could be more fun than going to the beach with the kids or hopping into the canoe for a paddle around the lake? But before you and your family

---

CHOOSING AND USING A PERSONAL FLOTATION DEVICE

•Always buy a US Coast Guard–approved personal flotation device (PFD). There are different types of PFDs for different water activities. Be sure to choose the right one for your needs.

•If you're buying a PFD for yourself, try it on first to see if it fits comfortably. It's a good idea to test it too. You can do this in shallow water by relaxing your body and letting your head tilt back. The PFD should keep your chin above water so that you can breathe easily.

•Be sure to buy your child a properly fitted PFD. Put it on your child and lift him by the shoulders. The PFD fits if his chin and ears don't slip through.

•Fasten all straps, zippers, and ties. Tuck in any loose ends so they won't get caught on anything.

•When your PFD feels stiff and no longer bounces back when you touch it, it's time for a new one.

•Take steps to ensure that your PFD is in good condition:

•Avoid crushing your PFD with heavy objects or by sitting or kneeling on it.

•After use, allow your PFD to dry thoroughly before putting it away. *DO NOT* use a direct heat source, such as a heater, to dry it.

•Store your PFD in a dry, well-ventilated place.

•Put your name on your PFD so that only you wear it. That way you'll know that your PFD will always fit and will be in good working order.

HOW TO SURVIVE IN COLD WATER

•For the signs and symptoms of hypothermia and how to treat it, see Hypothermia, page 117.

•Pull yourself onto a large floating object (if one is nearby) so that you can get as much of your body out of the water as possible.

•If you must remain in the water, use the heat escape lessening position (HELP)—draw your knees to your chest and cross your arms in front of you. Keep as quiet as possible. Be sure to keep your head and face out of cold water.

•If others are in the water with you, huddle together for warmth.

•*DO NOT* swim unless a boat, another person, or a floating object is within easy reach. Swimming will lower your body temperature even further.

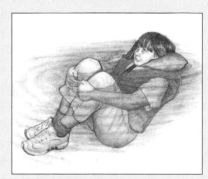

The HELP position.

make the splash, be sure you know and obey the basics of water and boating safety.

SAFETY GUIDELINES FOR CHILDREN

•*DO NOT* leave younger children alone near water. (For more information on home pool safety, see Safety Around the House and in the Garden, page 195).

•Enroll your child in swimming lessons at an early age. With these lessons, he will be better prepared to safely handle all types of water and boating situations.

•All children should wear a personal flotation device (PFD) when on docks or boats or while inner tubing.

•*DO NOT* rely on flotation devices, such as water wings or rafts, to keep your child safe in the water. A PFD should always be used.

•*DO NOT* leave a child alone near a body of frozen water.

SAFETY FOR TEENS AND ADULTS

•No one, not even adults, should swim alone.

•Adults and teens should wear a PFD on boats and while inner tubing.

•If you're driving a boat, stay well clear of marked swimming areas.

•If you're towing a water skier or someone in an inner tube or other device, designate one person to watch him at all times.

•Learn how to perform CPR (see page 12). Ideally, you should take a hands-on training course.

•Install propeller guards on all motor boats.

•*DO NOT* drink alcohol or take medications or drugs if you plan to swim or drive a boat.

GENERAL SAFETY GUIDELINES

•Make sure everyone follows the lifeguard's instructions and rules.

•If someone is in trouble in the water, perform a water rescue (see Drowning, page 84).

•*AVOID* falling into cold water, since water of less than 70°F puts you at risk of hypothermia (below-normal body temperature). If your body temperature gets too low, you can lose consciousness and drown. It's vital to learn how to survive if you fall into cold water (see page 213).

•*DO NOT* dive into an unknown lake, stream, or other body of water.

Be Safe When You Fish

For many people, fishing is a relaxing activity—a way to get away from it all. Still, there are some measures to keep in mind to make your fishing expedition a safe one.

•Tell a friend or relative about your fishing plans and when you'll return.

•Pack extra, warm clothes, rain gear, and a hat. Dress in layers. Take along sunscreen and insect repellent as well.

•Wear a PFD when you're in the boat. Make sure everyone else does too.

FISHHOOK INJURIES

Be especially careful handling fishhooks, which can easily pierce the skin. See pages 134 and 135 for how to treat a fishhook injury.

•Keep track of weather patterns. If a storm is approaching, get back to shore immediately. If there's no time, stay with the boat even if it capsizes. Most small boats can be righted. If this is not possible, climb onto the bottom of the boat that is above water and hang on. *DO NOT* attempt to swim to shore if the boat capsizes (see How to Survive in Cold Water, page 213).

•If you're fly fishing, take care not to cast too close to others. Be sure your footing is firm. If the current is too strong to maintain your balance, move to another area.

•Take a first aid kit with you. (See Home First Aid Kit, page 2).

•*DO NOT* drink alcohol while fishing.

SPORTS INJURIES

Sports are a great way for you and your family to be active together. You can have fun and stay fit, all at the same time. But bear in mind that injuries can happen. The good news is that most sports injuries can be prevented by using common sense and taking proper precautions, whenever you and your family are active.

Before You Play

•Get into shape before you begin your sport. Build up your fitness level gradually by setting reasonable goals—increase the length of your workout by no more than 10 percent per week. Follow a fitness program that includes strength training, flexibility and cardiovascular training. Even children, aged 7 and up, can engage in moderate strength training under adult supervision. Strong muscles mean less injury.

•Wear the proper attire. Most important is well-made, supportive footwear that is appropriate for the surface you'll be playing on. Clothing should suit the sport and the weather.

FOR MORE INFORMATION...

Professional medical organizations, such as the American Academy of Orthopaedic Surgeons, can provide information on sports injuries. For details, see page 256.

KNOW THE SCORE ON CONCUSSIONS

Everyone involved with athletes, particularly coaches and parents, should be familiar with the American Academy of Neurology's Guidelines on the Management of Concussion in Sports. These guidelines can help you properly assess a player's head injury and decide whether it's safe to send him back into the game. To obtain a copy, call the American Academy of Neurology at 651-695-1940 or go to www.guideline.gov (see also page 256).

•Buy and always wear protective equipment. Depending on the sport, you may need a helmet, protective eyewear, pads, or a mouthguard (see Mouthguards and Protective Eyewear Make Sense, below). Make sure this equipment fits properly and is comfortable.

•Always use good quality sporting equipment that is in good working order.

•Learn the skills needed for your sport, preferably from a trained professional. Improper technique can lead to injury.

•Inspect the area that you or your child will be playing on. Make sure it is free of trash, bottles, and other unsafe objects. Have holes, bumps, or other uneven surfaces fixed.

•Make sure your child's coach can recognize injuries and has a plan for handling injuries and emergencies, including a well-stocked first aid kit (see also Know the Score on Concussions).

•Always warm up before you play. A warm-up can include 5 minutes of brisk walking, followed by light,

MOUTHGUARDS AND PROTECTIVE EYEWEAR MAKE SENSE

Mouthguards and protective eyewear are important tools in your sports injury prevention kit and can prevent many facial, eye, and dental injuries.

PROTECTIVE EYEWEAR
•Eyeglass guards or protective eyewear should be used for all racquet sports, as well as baseball and ice hockey.
•Choose eye protection made of polycarbonate and make sure it meets ASTM impact standards.
•Remember that regular prescription eyeglasses and contact lenses don't protect against eye injuries from sports.

MOUTHGUARDS
There are three types of mouthguards:
•*Custom-made*: designed by your dentist from a cast made of your teeth
•*Mouth-formed*: also fitted by your dentist by shaping a soft guard to your teeth and allowing it to harden
•*Ready-made*: prefabricated from rubber or polyvinyl and sold at most sporting goods stores

Custom-made guards are more expensive but offer the best protection, particularly if you have braces or bridgework. Be sure *not* to wear removable dental work, such as retainers or dentures, when you play sports.

gentle stretches. Avoid bouncing movements while stretching.

When You Play

•Always drink plenty of fluids when you're active.

•Avoid strenuous exercise and activity on hot, humid days. Keep track of the weather (see below).

•If you walk or run at night outside, go with another person, wear reflective clothing, and keep to well-lit areas.

•Treat all sports injuries early. See Sprains and Strains (page 157), Dislocations (page 83), and Broken Bones (page 50).

•Cool down whenever you've finished your activity with smooth, gentle stretching and a slow walk around the block.

•*DO NOT* allow your child to exercise outside after dark.

•*DO NOT* exercise through pain. Listen to your body. If you feel pain, stop immediately and seek medical attention.

•*DO NOT* overtrain. Signs of overtraining include irritability, sleeping problems and weight loss. If you notice these signs, take a break from your regular exercise routine to rest and recover.

KEEP TRACK OF THE WEATHER WHEN YOU PLAY

IF IT BECOMES HOT

•Drink even more fluids than you think you need, both during and after the activity. Drink even if you're not thirsty. Plain water is usually best, although sports drinks are suitable when you're involved in strenuous exercise lasting more than an hour.

•Be sure to apply sunscreen and try to wear a hat.

•If you start to feel overheated, stop exercising immediately, get out of the sun, pour cool water on your head, and drink plenty of fluids. Learn the signs of heat exhaustion (see page 112) and heatstroke (see page 113) and how to treat these conditions.

•Salt tablets are not recommended and can cause problems if taken.

IF IT BECOMES COLD

•Put on extra layers of clothing and keep moving. Cold muscles are more prone to injury.

•*DO NOT* be a weekend-only exerciser. Thirty minutes of moderate exercise every day is far healthier than a weekend burst of activity.

SAFETY IN THE WORKPLACE

Since most of us spend a good part of our day in the workplace, ensuring that a work environment is safe makes good sense. There are many workplace guidelines that you and your coworkers can follow including to

•Use protection and safety equipment as needed.

•Learn how to perform CPR (see page 12) and to use an automated external defibrillator (for details, see page 21).

•Follow safe work procedures, such as the proper handling of chemicals or blood products.

•Know what to do in case of a fire or emergency and where to find fire extinguishers, first aid kits, and, if available, the first aid room or center.

VIOLENT WEATHER

Floods, tornadoes, hurricanes, and earthquakes are examples of violent weather in the United States. While you can't control Mother Nature, you can prepare for and handle some of the more extreme weather conditions that come your way.

Preparing for Violent Weather

•Be alert for storm watches, warnings, or advisories. Always obey evacuation orders.

•Ensure you are well stocked with food and bottled water that will last 72 hours.

•Check your flashlight, batteries, and fire extinguishers.

•Secure all antennas, satellite dishes, and other outside objects.

•Bring in outdoor furniture and turn off external gas lines.

FOR MORE INFORMATION...

The National Weather Service Web site is a good source for weather information and safety tips. See page 258.

•Trim trees that are too close to power lines. Have your roof inspected and prepared.

•Ensure your car is in good working order and has a full tank of gas.

•Review maps and evacuation routes and check that your first aid kit is well stocked.

•Buy a battery-powered radio.

•Stock up on essential medications.

IN CASE YOU ARE FORCED OUT OF YOUR HOME, ALSO HAVE READY

•Warm clothes, footwear, and gloves for the entire family

•Alternative light sources, such as candles and waterproof matches

•Blankets, tent, sleeping bags

•Tool kit

•Copies of essential documents and extra cash, including coins for a payphone; your fully charged cell phone, if you have one

---

DID YOU KNOW...

By keeping trees that are close to power lines trimmed, you can reduce the risk of an electrical outage during a storm.

When Bad Weather Strikes

FLOODS

•If your car stalls, get out immediately and walk to higher ground.

•Exercise caution at night, when flood waters are more difficult to see.

•Flood water will be filled with sewage and other garbage. *DO NOT* eat food exposed to flood waters and don't drink flood water unless you treat it with purifying tablets, filters, or mechanical purifiers. Have your well water flushed and checked before drinking it.

•Wear pants and long sleeves to avoid being cut by debris in flood water.

•*DO NOT* try to walk or drive through flood waters. Go around if possible and seek higher ground.

TORNADOES AND HURRICANES

•If you're at home, go to the basement or a storm shelter. Otherwise, huddle in the bathroom, closet, or interior bedroom, away from exterior walls, and duck under a sturdy table or other heavy piece of furniture. Hold the table with one hand and protect your head with the other. Move with the table if necessary.

•Stay there until the storm passes.

•If you're in a mobile home, trailer, or car during a hurricane, head inland and avoid low-lying areas.

•If you're in a mobile home, trailer, or car when a tornado strikes, get out and find the lowest ground you can, like a ditch or other depression. Lie flat with your arms over your head.

EARTHQUAKES

•Duck under a sturdy table or other heavy piece of furniture. Hold the table with one hand and protect your head with the other. Move with the table if necessary.

•If there is no table or other suitable furniture, sit on the floor against an interior wall well away from windows or tall furniture. Hold this position until the shaking stops.

•If you're outside, keep away from trees, buildings, or downed electrical wires.

•If you're driving, move to the shoulder and stop, well away from overpasses, power lines, or tall buildings.

•Be prepared for aftershocks.

•*DO NOT* run outside or use the stairs or any elevators.

BLIZZARDS

•If you're at home, stay there until the storm passes.

•If you get caught in a blizzard in your car and you're unable to drive, stay in the car unless you're very close to a house or other building. If you have a cellular phone, call for help. Run the engine periodically to keep the car warm, but be sure to leave the window open slightly to remove poisonous fumes. Leave your emergency flashers on to let others know you are there. Move your arms and legs now and then to help yourself stay awake and keep warm.

LIGHTNING

•If you're indoors, stay there. Unplug your computer, TV, and VCR, and stay off the telephone. *AVOID* sources of water, such as the shower, faucets, or sinks. Stay away from the fireplace, windows, and open doors.

•If you're walking outside and not near a building or your car, stay low and find shelter under a group of *short* trees. If you're in an open field, kneel or squat. *DO NOT* lie flat. If you are with others, do not group together; spread out. Stay well away from tall trees, hills, open fields, swimming pools or other bodies of water, and metal objects such as umbrellas, golf clubs, fishing poles, boat masts, and utility poles.

•If you're in a boat or in the water, get to shore immediately.

•Your car (as long as it has a hard top) is a safe place to be, although if visibility is poor, pull over until the storm blows over.

When the Violent Weather Has Passed

•Turn off the gas supply at the meter if you smell any gas.

•Check for any injuries, and provide first aid.

•Assist others, especially the young, elderly, disabled, or injured.

•Listen to the radio for instructions.

•Inspect your home for damage.

•*DO NOT* use the telephone unless it's a life-threatening emergency—in order to avoid overloading telephone systems.

PLAYING IT SAFE IN THE WORLD

SAFETY PREPARATION FOR TERRORIST ATTACKS

Terrorist attacks can happen anywhere, at any time, not only abroad but in our own country as well. While it's important to keep the threat of terrorism in perspective, it's equally important to be aware of potential threats and to prepare yourself and your family for unexpected emergencies.

Terrorism can take many forms, including

•*Biological attacks:* the deliberate release of germs or other substances that can make people sick if inhaled, eaten, or entered through a cut in the skin. There are three types of biological agents: bacteria (such as anthrax), viruses (such as smallpox), and toxins or poisonous substances found in, and taken from, living plants or animals.

•*Chemical attacks:* the deliberate release of toxic gases, liquids, or solids that can poison people and their surrounding environment.

•*Radioactive attacks:* the deliberate detonation of radioactive material. For terrorists, the most likely radioactive weapon is a "dirty bomb," a conventional bomb combined with radioactive material. It is designed to spread dangerous amounts of this material over a general area. The damage from a dirty bomb is both immediate and delayed, due to the risk of spread or contamination after the impact of the initial explosion.

How To Handle Suspicious Packages

Everyone should know how to recognize and handle suspicious packages and envelopes. Try to identify suspicious envelopes or packages by:

•Unsuitable or unexpected labeling, such as too much postage, no return address, threatening language, misspelling of common words

WHAT YOU NEED TO KNOW ABOUT ANTHRAX

Anthrax is a serious yet rare disease caused by a bacterium—a tiny, free-living organism-that forms spores which allow it to reproduce. This disease is most often found in wild and domestic animals, such as antelope and cattle, but it can also affect people who have been exposed to the spores, usually from infected animals or their tissue. Anthrax has been used as a biological terrorist weapon—in 2001, several people in the United States were exposed to anthrax from letters that were deliberately filled with anthrax spores made into white powder.

HOW IT SPREADS

People are most commonly infected through a cut in the skin (cutaneous anthrax). They can also come into contact with anthrax by eating meat (intestinal anthrax) or by inhaling the spores (inhalation anthrax), which causes the most serious, usually fatal form of the disease. It is extremely unlikely for anthrax to spread from one person to another.

SIGNS AND SYMPTOMS

Signs and symptoms of anthrax usually show up within 7 days of exposure and vary depending on the form of the disease:

•*Cutaneous anthrax:* begins with an itchy bump (like an insect bite) that, within 1 to 2 days, develops into a fluid-filled blister and then into a painless, open sore 1 to 3 cm in diameter with a black area in the middle.

•*Intestinal anthrax:* nausea, vomiting, loss of appetite, and fever appear first, followed by abdominal pain, vomiting of blood, and severe diarrhea.

•*Inhalation anthrax:* begins with symptoms of the common cold, which may progress to severe breathing problems and shock (see pages 47 and 146).

TREATMENT

Anthrax can be treated with antibiotics. Treatment is most effective when antibiotics are given at the early stages of infection.

PREVENTION

An anthrax vaccine can prevent the disease. However, it is not available to the general public at this time.

•Appearance, such as unusual stains, odors or discoloration; protruding wires; or aluminium foil

•Other suspicious signs, for example, seems overly heavy

•If a package or envelope appears suspicious

  •*DO NOT* open it or shake the contents.

  •Place it in a container (such as a plastic bag). If a container isn't available, cover the package or envelope with anything available (such as a cardboard or paper).

- *DO NOT* touch, sniff, or look closely at the package or envelope or any contents that may have spilled out.
- Alert others. Leave the area, close any doors, and keep everyone away.
- Wash hands with soap and water.
- Alert a supervisor, security officer, or local law enforcement official.
- If possible, compile a list of those in the area and those who may have handled the package or envelope, and give this list to public health and law enforcement officials.

WHAT YOU NEED TO KNOW ABOUT SMALLPOX

Smallpox is a serious, sometimes fatal disease caused by the variola virus. After a worldwide vaccination program, smallpox was declared eradicated in 1980. However, the smallpox virus still exists in some laboratories and could potentially be used as a biological weapon.

HOW IT SPREADS
Direct and lengthy face-to-face contact with an infected person is usually needed to spread smallpox from one person to another. Smallpox can also be spread through infected bodily fluids or contaminated bedding, clothing, and other objects. Only in rare cases has smallpox been spread by the virus being carried through the air in an enclosed space (such as buses and buildings). It is not known to be spread by insects or animals.

SIGNS AND SYMPTOMS
After a person is exposed to smallpox, it takes 7 to 17 days for symptoms to develop. During this period, the person feels healthy and cannot pass on the virus. Fever, head and body aches, and vomiting are usually the first symptoms to appear. These symp-

toms are very similar to those associated with the flu and other viral illnesses. What sets smallpox apart is a rash that develops, spreads, and progresses to raised bumps and pus-filled blisters. After about 3 weeks, the blisters crust, scab, and fall off, leaving a pitted scar. An infected person is most contagious from the time the rash appears to when the last scab falls off.

TREATMENT
There is no proven treatment for smallpox, although people can be helped with intensive, supportive hospital care. Most people with smallpox recover, although many will have permanent scars, especially on their face. Blindness may also occur.

PREVENTION
The smallpox vaccine is the only way to prevent the disease. The American public has not been routinely vaccinated since 1972, after the disease was officially wiped out. However, the 2001 terrorist attacks prompted the American government to order enough smallpox vaccinations to immunize all people in the event that the

These and other steps for identifying and handling suspicious envelopes or packages are provided by the Centers for Disease Control and Prevention (CDC) at www.bt.cdc.gov. (See Resources section, page 246 for other CDC contact information)

How You Can Prepare for Potential Terrorist Attacks

There are simple, common-sense steps you can take to ready yourself and your loved ones for the possibility of terrorist attacks, such as developing a family emergency plan, assembling an emergency supply kit, and preparing for sheltering in your

---

WHAT YOU NEED TO KNOW ABOUT SMALLPOX *(continued)*

virus were used as a biological weapon. (This has been done by the CDC's National Pharmaceutical Stockpile NPS Program, see Stockpile Stands Ready, page 226.) At this time, the smallpox vaccine is not available to the general public, but certain healthcare professionals who would respond to a smallpox emergency are being vaccinated.

VACCINE SAFETY

The smallpox vaccine is safe for most people, who usually experience mild reactions (such as a sore arm or fever). For a small percentage (about 1 per thousand people) the reactions can be more severe. In rare cases (about 14 to 52 per million people), life- threatening reactions may occur. To help prevent these complications, certain groups of people should consult with their physician *before* proceeding with vaccination even if they have been exposed to the smallpox virus:

•People allergic to anything in the vaccine (polymyxin B, streptomycin, chlortetracycline, neomycin)

•People with present or previous skin conditions, especially eczema or atopic dermatitis

•People with weakened immune systems (such as those who have received a transplant, are HIV positive, or are receiving cancer treatment)

•Pregnant and breastfeeding women

•Children under 12 months of age

•People currently using steroid drops in their eyes

•People diagnosed with a heart condition (with or without symptoms)

•People who have three or more of the following: high blood pressure, high blood cholesterol, diabetes, high blood sugar, or a first degree relative (parent, sibling, or child) with a heart condition before the age of 50, and/or people who currently smoke cigarettes

For more detailed information about smallpox, visit www.cdc.gov/smallpox.

STOCKPILE STANDS READY

Since 1999, the CDC's National Pharmaceutical Stockpile program has created a national inventory of lifesaving medications, vaccines (including smallpox), antidotes, and medical supplies and equipment. These resources are stored at strategic locations across the country to ensure that they are available and accessible to all American civilians in the event of a biological or chemical terrorist attack.

home. The government is preparing as well (see Stockpile Stands Ready).

DEVELOPING A FAMILY EMERGENCY PLAN

Developing a family emergency plan is an important first step in preparing for potential terrorist attacks as well as other disasters:

•Find out about the emergency response plans in your community, particularly where you work and at your children's day care or school.

•Discuss potential emergencies with your family—how to handle them, and what you would need.

•Develop a communications plan—identify one meeting place near your home (such as a tree) and another away from your neighborhood in case you can't return home.

•Pick a relative or friend who lives outside your area to call, if necessary. An out-of-state contact may be better, as it may be easier to place a long-distance call than a local call. Be sure each member of your family over age 8 always has coins or a pre-paid phone card. Make sure children are properly trained on how to use a pay phone.

•Mark two escape routes from each room on your home's floor plan.

•Post emergency phone numbers by the phone, and teach your children how to call 911.

•If you, or a member of your family, have a disability or special need, make arrangements for disaster warnings and assistance for sheltering. Special assistance may be provided in your community (for example, the office of emergency services or the fire department). Call these resources for more information.

EMERGENCY SUPPLY KITS

An emergency supply kit is vital for keeping you and your family safe and healthy if a terrorist attack occurs. According to the US Department of Homeland Security, a well-stocked kit includes provisions for water, food, and clean air, as well as basic emergency supplies, and a first aid kit (see page 2). It should have supplies for 3 days, although you may consider storing additional supplies so that your kit can last up to 2 weeks.

Preparing an Emergency Supply Kit

Your emergency supply kit should be kept in a designated area and be ready to take with you in case you have to leave your home quickly. Be sure your family knows where the kit is kept.

WATER

•Store at least 3-day's supply of water per person in clean plastic containers, such as soft drink bottles. Each person will need approximately 1 gallon of water per day for drinking and sanitation, although more may be needed if there are children, nursing mothers or sick people present, or if you live in a warmer climate.

•Rinse water containers with a diluted bleach solution (1 part bleach to 10 parts water).

•If you have well or public water that has not been treated, treat water (according to directions from your public health service or water provider) before storing it.

•Change stored water every 6 months.

FOOD

•Store at least 3-day's supply of nonperishable food that needs no refrigeration, preparation, or cooking and little or no water (for example, ready-to-eat canned meat, fruits, or vegetables, peanut butter, crackers, nuts, nonperishable pasteurized milk, and infant food, if necessary). Try to choose foods your family will like.

•Store cans in a dry, cool place and boxed foods in tightly closed plastic or metal containers.

•Mark the date on each food item. Replace items every 6 months. Discard any cans that become swollen, dented, or corroded.

CLEAN AIR

Store supplies that will create a barrier between yourself and any contamination.

•Face masks (see Face Masks Guidelines, page

233) or dense-weave cotton material that will snugly cover your nose and mouth (be sure to consider the right fit for each member of your family).

•Heavyweight plastic bags or plastic sheeting, duct tape, and scissors—these supplies can be used to tape up windows, doors, and air vents if you need to seal off a room (see Sheltering, page 229).

BASIC SUPPLIES
•Flashlight
•Battery-powered radio
•Extra batteries
•Waterproof matches or standard matches in a waterproof container
•Manual can opener, utility knife
•Plastic utensils, plates, and paper cups
•Plastic storage container
•Small fire extinguisher (ABC type)
•Pliers, shut-off wrench (to turn off household gas and water)
•Map of the local area
•Whistle
•Signal flare
•Tube tent
•One complete change of warm clothing and shoes for each person
•Sleeping bag or warm blanket for each person

HOME FIRST AID KIT
See page 2 for a description of the contents of a home first aid kit.

SANITATION
•Toilet paper, paper towels, moist towelettes
•Personal hygiene items (such as toothpaste, toothbrush, deodorants, feminine protection)
•Plastic garbage bags, ties
•Plastic bucket with tight lid
•Household chlorine bleach, which can be used as a disinfectant or, in an emergency, to purify water-mix 16 drops of regular household liquid bleach

with 1 gallon of water. Avoid bleaches that are scented, color-safe, or have added cleaners.

IMPORTANT DOCUMENTS AND SPECIALTY ITEMS

•Insurance policies, bank account records, personal identification (store in waterproof container)

•Emergency contact list and phone numbers

•Cash or traveler's checks, change

•Extra set of car and house keys

•Prescription medications (with list of these medications and doses). Be sure to ask your doctor how to properly store medications. Always check expiration dates and update all of your medications when necessary.

•Contact lenses and supplies; extra eyeglasses

•Be sure to plan for the needs of infants, disabled persons, and pets.

For more information on Emergency/Disaster Plans and Kits, visit www.ready.gov, or *Are You Ready? A Guide to Citizen Preparedness* by the Federal Emergency Management Agency (FEMA), available at www.fema.gov/areyouready.

SHELTERING

In the event of an emergency, taking shelter may be essential for protecting yourself and your family. Sheltering may be in-place (taking shelter at the location where you are when disaster strikes) or mass sheltering (taking shelter in a facility with others who evacuate during a disaster).

In-Place Sheltering

In some emergency situations, it will be best for you and your family to seek in-place sheltering (particularly if advised to do so by the authorities). In fact, it may be a matter of survival. To prepare for in-place sheltering:

•Identify an internal, windowless room at your home or work where you can take shelter.

•Store your Emergency Supply Kit (see page 226)

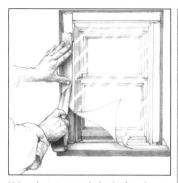

Using duct tape and plastic sheeting to seal a window.

in or near this room—the duct tape and plastic sheeting in your kit will let you seal the room by taping up windows, doors, and air vents. To save time, measure and cut the sheeting in advance.

•Consider placing a portable air filter with a HEPA filter in the room to help remove contaminants, if necessary.

•If you need to remain in the shelter for an extended period of time, you will have to consider important issues such as managing water and food supplies and assembling an emergency toilet. Detailed information on preparing for and implementing long-term in-place sheltering can be obtained in *Are You Ready? A Guide to Citizen Preparedness* by the Federal Emergency Management Agency, available at www.fema.gov/areyouready.

REDUCING YOUR RISK OF COMMUNICABLE DISEASE

In your home environment, you may be exposed to locally occurring viruses and bacteria that can cause communicable disease (disease that can be spread, directly or indirectly, from one person to another). In addition, there are the communicable diseases brought home by international travelers—a growing phenomenon as increasing numbers of people travel greater distances for professional, recreational, and humanitarian purposes.

As a result, our world continues to experience outbreaks of "old" communicable diseases like influenza (flu) and new ones such as Sudden Acute Respiratory Syndrome (SARS). It's important to understand that these outbreaks are independent of potential terrorist attacks using biological agents (see Safety Preparation for Terrorist Attacks, pages 222 to 230).

Ongoing global efforts address infectious disease outbreaks and try to contain, eradicate, and prevent them. What's more, there are many things you can do to protect yourself and your family from being exposed to, and passing on, communicable diseases.

Practice Good Hygiene

The first line of defense against many communicable diseases is good hand hygiene. The Centers for Disease Control and Prevention (CDC) recommends frequent handwashing with soap and water. Ideally, you should use warm, soapy water and lather for 20 seconds. If your hands are not visibly dirty, you can use an alcohol-based handrub or waterless soap as an alternative.

•Use household disinfectant to clean doorknobs, phones, and other items (such as children's toys) that might have saliva or other fluids from the nose, mouth, or eyes on them.

•Promptly throw away any tissues or other articles that have contact with your nose, mouth, or eyes.

•Do not share personal items (such as drinking cups, eating utensils, and toothbrushes) with others.

Consider Vaccines

Vaccines are usually the best way to prevent communicable diseases. There are some vaccines that you should get, particularly if you are traveling. (See Safety Preparation Before Traveling, page 199.) And don't forget about a yearly flu vaccine—it's very effective for preventing the flu and is particularly important for people at high risk of developing complications (for details, see Flu Shots, page 233).

Influenza

Influenza (flu) is a contagious disease caused by the influenza virus. It affects the respiratory tract (lungs, nose, and throat). The flu most commonly occurs from late December to March and affects about 10% to 20% of Americans every year. You may be surprised to learn that about 36,000 Americans die every year from complications of the flu (such as pneumonia, dehydration, or worsening of chronic conditions such as asthma). The people at highest risk for these complications are the very young, very old, and those with severe immunocompromising illnesses (such as HIV or AIDS).

HOW IT SPREADS

When a person with the flu coughs, sneezes, or speaks, the virus is released into the air. Other people become sick when they inhale the virus. It can also be spread if you touch a surface with the virus on it (for example, a door handle) and then touch your nose or mouth.

SIGNS AND SYMPTOMS

Fever, body aches, headache, tiredness (sometimes extreme), dry cough, sore throat, and nasal congestion are the most common flu symptoms, which generally appear 1 to 4 days after the virus has entered the body. A person with the flu is contagious 1 day before symptoms appear. Adults can pass on the virus for 3 to 7 days after symptoms start, while children can pass it on for longer than 7 days.

TREATMENT

Once you have the flu, drink plenty of fluids, take medication to treat your symptoms, and *AVOID* alcohol and tobacco. Antiviral drugs (prescribed by a doctor) can reduce the duration of the flu if given within the first few days of the illness, but they can't cure it.

PREVENTION

The best method of prevention is the flu vaccine ("shot"). Studies of healthy people have shown the flu shot to be 70% to 90% effective. It is vital to have the flu shot every year—flu viruses are constantly changing, so the vaccine must be changed every year to keep up with new strains of the virus. Remember that the flu shot is made from flu viruses that have been inactivated (killed), so it can't cause the flu.

FLU SHOTS

The CDC recommends a yearly flu shot for

- People at high risk for complications
  - People over 50 years of age
  - Residents of nursing homes and other long-term care facilities
  - Adults and children over 6 months of age with chronic heart or lung conditions (such as asthma)
  - Adults and children over 6 months of age who have regular medical care for metabolic diseases (such as diabetes), chronic kidney disease, or weakened immune systems (caused by medicine or infection with disease, such as HIV or AIDS)
  - Children and teenagers aged 6 months to 18 years on long-term aspirin therapy
  - Women who will be more than 3 months pregnant during the flu season
- People who can give the flu to high-risk people (listed above)
  - Doctors, nurses, and other employees in hospitals and doctors' offices

- Employees of nursing homes and other long-term care facilities in direct contact with residents
- Employees of assisted living and other residences of high-risk people
- People who provide home care to high-risk people
- Household members (including children) of high-risk people

- Anyone else in the population who wants to reduce their chances of getting the flu

Flu shots are *NOT* recommended for

- People with a severe allergy to hens' eggs

- People with a previous severe reaction to the flu shot

- People who previously developed Guillain-Barre syndrome, a disorder in which the body's immune system attacks peripheral nerves (those outside the brain and spinal cord) in the 6 weeks following a flu shot

Face Mask Guidelines

Face masks help to protect you not only from biological agents used in terrorist attacks (see page 222) but also from communicable diseases. The general public is not always advised to wear face masks (see What You Need to Know About SARS, page 235). However, if you do decide to buy them, here are some important tips from the Good Housekeeping Institute. Remember—not all masks are the same.

CHOOSE THE RIGHT MASK

- The best mask is a filtering facepiece mask. Sometimes called an N95, N99, or N100 mask, they are 95%, 99%, and 99.7% effective, respectively, at filtering small particles from the air.

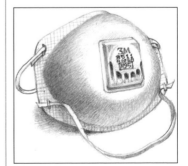

N95 face mask

These masks are approved by the National Institute of Occupational Safety and Health (NIOSH), which means they've been tested to ensure that tiny particles won't pass through.

•Surgical and "comfort" masks sold at drug and hardware stores do not provide enough protection from viruses that are transmitted through saliva and mucus when an infected person sneezes or coughs. Studies have found that these masks may only prevent 30% to 40% of particles from being inhaled.

TEST THE FIT

•An effective mask should feel snug on your face. Men should shave their beards for better protection. Look for a filtering facepiece that's molded and has inserts over the nose.

•You can also check the fit by exhaling; if air escapes over the top (by your nose), look for a different model or another size. Most masks come in small, medium, and large sizes.

LOOK FOR AN EXHALATION VALVE

•An exhalation valve is a small circle on the front of the mask. If you plan to wear the mask for several hours (for example, on an overseas flight), this valve lets your moist breath escape, minimizing skin irritation.

BUY DISPOSABLE MASKS IN BULK

•Disposable masks are designed to be worn only once (up to 8 hours, depending on the environment) and should be thrown away immediately after using them.

•If you think you've been exposed to a communicable disease (such as SARS) while wearing a mask, dispose of it in a sealed plastic bag and replace the mask with a new one. Wash your hands after handling the mask and contact your doctor immediately.

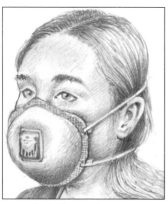
Proper fit of a face mask.

SEVERE ACUTE RESPIRATORY SYNDROME

Severe acute respiratory syndrome (SARS) is a serious, sometimes fatal disease that affects the respiratory tract (lungs, nose, and throat). Cases of SARS have been reported in Asia, North America, and Europe. In the United States, most cases have occurred among travelers returning home from countries affected by SARS, and there is no evidence that the disease is spreading more widely. Scientists believe that SARS is caused by a previously unknown virus in the coronavirus family. The most effective treatment for SARS is unknown. However, people can be helped with fluids as well as pain and fever medication.

It appears that SARS mainly spreads by close person-to-person contact including:

•People living in the same house with, or caring for, a person with SARS

•Those who have direct contact with infectious droplets (released when the sick person coughs or sneezes) or bodily fluids of a person with SARS

It is also possible that this disease may spread in other ways that are currently not known.

RECOGNIZING SYMPTOMS OF ILLNESS

SARS often begins with a fever over 100.4°F. Other symptoms can include headache, body aches and discomfort, and mild respiratory problems. After 2 to 7 days, a dry cough and breathing difficulties may develop. It is believed that people infected with SARS are most contagious when they show the symptoms of the disease, although it is unknown how long before or after these symptoms appear that the disease can be passed on.

PREVENTION POINTERS

•Frequent hand washing is the best way to protect yourself and your family (for details, see page 231).

•Avoid touching your eyes, nose, and mouth when your hands are unclean.

•Encourage people to cover their nose and mouth with a tissue when coughing or sneezing.

•The CDC does not recommend the routine wearing of a face mask for the general public, although if you do decide to wear masks, buy wisely (see Face Mask Guidelines, page 233).

Note: More stringent preventive measures are recommended for people who have or live with a person who has SARS, care for people with SARS, or are traveling to areas with SARS.

For more information on SARS, go to www.cdc.gov/ncidod/sars and www.who.int.csr.sars.en.

Stay Up-to-Date

By arming yourself with accurate, up-to-date information, you can get a realistic picture of emerging communicable diseases relevant to you and your family and what you can do about them. The Centers for Disease Control and Prevention

(CDC) provides the latest public information on these diseases. Visit the CDC's National Center for Infectious Diseases at www.cdc.gov/ncidod. Specific information on travel-related diseases and outbreaks is available at the Web site www.cdc.gov/travel. You can also refer to the Safety Preparation Before Traveling section on pages 199 and 200 of this book.

RESOURCES

FIRST AID COURSES

American Red Cross
Public Inquiry Office
2025 East Street NW
Washington, DC 20006
Phone: 202-303-4498
Web site: www.redcross.org

The American Red Cross provides first aid training, community programs, and courses for children, adults, emergency response professionals, and instructors. It even offers pet first aid. Contact your local Red Cross chapter for information about courses and programs.

Emergency Cardiovascular Care
American Heart Association (AHA)
National Center
7272 Greenville Avenue
Dallas, TX 75231
Phone: 800-AHA-USA1 (800-242-8721)
Web site: www.americanheart.org

Its Web site has basic information on emergency cardiovascular care, such as CPR and automated external defibrillators, as well as the locations of local emergency cardiac care classes and AHA branches.

National Safety Council
1121 Spring Lake Drive
Itasca, IL 60143
Phone: 630-285-1121 or
800-621-7619 (for Council Chapters and Divisions)
Web site: www.nsc.org

The National Safety Council offers first aid and CPR courses.

GENERAL RESOURCES

American Academy of Pediatrics (AAP)
National Headquarters
141 Northwest Point Boulevard
Elk Grove Village, IL 60007
Phone: 847-434-4000
Web site: www.aap.org

The AAP provides comprehensive information for parents of children from birth to age 21. Topics covered include car safety, immunization, injury prevention, child abuse, water safety, allergies, croup, and much more.

US Consumer Product Safety Commission (CPSC)
Washington, DC 20207
Consumer Hotline: 800-638-2772
800-638-8270 (TTY)
Phone: 301-504-6816
Web site: www.cpsc.gov

The CPSC offers information on a wide range of safety-related issues, including carbon monoxide poisoning, fires and burns, safety barrier guidelines for home pools, car safety seats, product recalls, and much more.

RESOURCES BY TOPIC

AIDS

See HIV/AIDS & Hepatitis, page 251

ALCOHOL AND DRUG ABUSE

Alcoholics Anonymous (AA)
PO Box 459
Grand Central Station
New York, NY 10163
Phone: 212-870-3400
or look in the phone book for your local branch.
Web site: www.aa.org

AA is a group that helps its members achieve and maintain sobriety. Information about AA and how to join can be found on the Web site or by calling your local chapter.

Al-Anon/Alateen
Family Group Headquarters
1600 Corporate Landing Parkway
Virginia Beach, VA 23454
Phone: 888-425-2666
Web site: www.al-anon.org

Al-Anon/Alateen is a worldwide organization that offers a self-help recovery program for families and friends of alcoholics, whether or not the alcoholic seeks help or even acknowledges a drinking problem. You can find a meeting by calling the toll-free line or by accessing its online state directory.

Center for Substance Abuse Treatment
Substance Abuse and Mental Health Services
Administration
Room 12-105 Parklawn Building
5600 Fishers Lane
Rockville, MD 20857
Referral Helplines:
800-662-HELP (800-662-4357)
800-662-9832 (Spanish)
800-228-0427 (TTY)
Web site: www.samhsa.gov/csat/csat.htm

The Center for Substance Abuse Treatment is a referral service and national directory of drug abuse and alcoholism treatment and prevention programs.

National Clearinghouse for Alcohol and Drug Information
PO Box 2345
Rockville, MD 20847
Phone: 800-729-6686
800-487-4889 (TDD)
301-468-2600 (local callers)
Web site: www.health.org

Here you can obtain answers to your questions about alcohol, tobacco, and drugs.

National Institute on Alcohol Abuse and Alcoholism (NIAAA)
National Institutes of Health (NIH)
6000 Executive Boulevard—Willco Building
Bethesda, MD 20892
Phone: 301-496-4000 (NIH switchboard)
Web site: www.niaaa.nih.gov

Through the NIAAA, you can find details on research conducted on the causes, consequences, treatments, and prevention of alcoholism and alcohol-related problems. A useful FAQ (frequently asked questions) section on drug and alcohol abuse is included on the Web site.

ALLERGY AND ASTHMA

American Academy of Allergy, Asthma and Immunology
611 East Wells Street
Milwaukee, WI 53202
Phone: 800-822-2762
Web site: www.aaaai.org

A wide range of patient education materials on allergy and asthma are available on the Web site or by calling the number listed above. You can obtain names of allergy and asthma specialists in your area through their Physician Referral Directory.

Asthma and Allergy Network, Mothers of Asthmatics
2751 Prosperity Avenue, Suite 150
Fairfax, VA 22031
Phone: 800-878-4403 or
703-641-9595
Web site: www.aanma.org

This resource offers news, tips, and publications on asthma and allergy. On the Web site, you will find a listing of physicians (by name or location) who are members of this network as well as details of outreach services in communities across the country.

Allergy, Asthma & Immunology Online
http://allergy.mcg.edu

This site is an online source of information and news on allergy and asthma from the American College of Allergy, Asthma & Immunology (ACAAI). An allergist locator is also available.

AUTOMOBILE SAFETY

American Automobile Association Foundation for Traffic Safety
607 14th Streeet NW
Suite 201
Washington, DC 20005
Phone: 202-638-5944 or
800-305-SAFE (800-305-7233) for order
    fulfillment
Web site: www.aaafoundation.org

The AAA Foundation for Traffic Safety has information for everyone who uses the road, young and old, pedestrian and driver. Brochures are available on a range of driving-related topics including road rage and older drivers. To reach your local AAA club, which also provides safety information, go to www.aaa.com, which will direct you to the Web site of your local branch of AAA.

National Highway Traffic Safety Administration (NHTSA)
400 7th Street SW
Washington, DC 20590
Phone: 202-366-9550
Auto Safety Hotline: 888-DASH-2-DOT
(888-327-4236)
Web site: www.nhtsa.dot.gov

The NHTSA offers information on air bags, auto safety, car recalls, child passenger safety, and much more. You can also lodge vehicle complaints and problems through the NHTSA.

National Safety Council
1121 Spring Lake Drive
Itasca, IL 60143
Phone: 630-285-1121 or
800-621-7619 (for Council Chapters and Divisions)
Web site: www.nsc.org

Through the National Safety Council, you can find out about air bags, seat belts, and safety laws, as well as details on defensive driving courses and a list of training agency locations.

BICYCLING AND IN-LINE SKATING

American Society for Testing and Materials (ASTM)
100 Barr Harbor Drive
West Conshohocken, PA 19428

Phone: 610-832-9585
Web site: www.astm.org

Through the ASTM you can order standards on protective headgear, helmets for mountain biking, bicycle helmets for infants and toddlers, and mounting of child carriers and safety specifications on stationary exercise bikes.

Bicycle Helmet Safety Institute
4611 7th Street South
Arlington, VA 22204
Phone: 703-486-0100
Web site: www.bhsi.org

The Bicycle Helmet Safety Institute has useful online information, including a consumer's guide to bicycle helmets, standards, helmet and injury statistics, and helmet laws.

International Inline Skating Association (IISA)
105 South 7th Street
Wilmington, NC 28401
Phone: 910-762-7004
Web site: www.iisa.org

Online resources at the IISA cover learning to skate, rules of the road, health benefits, and safety data. On this site, you can also find a certified instructor near you.

Snell Memorial Foundation
3628 Madison Avenue, Suite 11
North Highlands, CA 95660
Phone: 916-331-5073 or 888-SNELL99 (888-763-5599)
Web site: www.smf.org

Snell sets, maintains, and upgrades helmet standards and tests helmets at its testing facility. You can obtain certified product lists, helmet standards, brochures, videos, stickers, pins, and other public

NOTES

safety information by calling Snell or visiting its Web site.

CAMPING

American Camping Association (ACA), Inc.
5000 State Road 67 N
Martinsville, IN 46151
Phone: 765-342-8456
Web site: http://www.acacamps.org

The ACA provides a database of over 2,000 ACA-accredited camps. ACA accreditation identifies those programs that offer a solid foundation of health, safety, and program quality.

Camping USA
Web site: www.camping-usa.com

Camping USA provides information such as checklists for camping supplies, campground directories, listings of special events around the country, and links to other camping resources.

National Park Service Headquarters
National Park Service Public Health Program
1849 C Street NW
Washington, DC 20240
Phone: 202-565-1120
Web site: http://www.nps.gov/public_health/

The National Park Service Public Health Program is responsible for protecting the health of approximately 270 million annual visitors to US national park facilities. This agency provides information and public health guidance on topics such as drinking water guidelines and food-, water-, insect-, and animal-borne diseases. The Web site also directs visitors to other important public health sites.

CHILD ABUSE

Childhelp USA National Headquarters
15757 N. 78th Street
Scottsdale, AZ 85260
Phone: 480-922-8212
Hotline: 800-4-A-CHILD (800-422-4453)
800-2-A-CHILD (800-222-4453) (TDD)
Web site: www.childhelpusa.org

Childhelp USA has a 24-hour-a-day toll-free line for anyone to call about child abuse, parenting, adult survivor abuse, or family violence issues. Through its hotline, you have access to trained professionals who provide counseling, information, and referral services.

National Center on Shaken Baby Syndrome (NCSBS)
2955 Harrison Boulevard, Room 102
Ogden, CT 84403
Phone: 888-273-0071 or 801-627-3399
Web site: www.dontshake.com

The National Center on Shaken Baby Syndrome (NCBS) is a good source for facts on Shaken Baby Syndrome (SBS), prevention tips, and information on infant brain injury. The Web site has a range of resources for parents and family members of syndrome survivors and victims and provides links to related sites on child abuse.

Parents Anonymous
National Office
675 W. Foothill Boulevard, Suite 220
Claremont, CA 91711
Phone: 909-621-6184
Web site: www.parentsanonymous.org

Parents Anonymous is a national network of community-based groups that help parents learn new skills and transform behaviors, attitudes, and actions. For information about activities and a 24-hour hotline in your state for immediate assistance to parents in need, contact the national organization above.

COMMUNICABLE DISEASES

Centers for Disease Control and Prevention (CDC)—National Center for Infectious Diseases
Office of Health Communication
National Center for Infectious Diseases
Centers for Disease Control and Prevention
Mailstop C-14
1600 Clifton Road
Atlanta, GA 30333
CDC Public Response Hotline:
Phone: 888-246-2675
888-246-2857 (Spanish)
866-874-2646 (TTY)
Web site: www.cdc.gov/ncidod

Through the CDC's National Center for Infectious Diseases, you can have access to the latest information and recommendations on emerging and long-standing communicable diseases.

World Health Organization
Regional Office for the Americas
525 23rd Street NW
Washington, DC 20037
Phone: 202-974-3000
Web site: www.who.int/en/

The World Health Organization provides current information on disease outbreaks, emergencies, and traveler's health.

DIABETES

American Diabetes Association
1701 North Beauregard Street
Alexandria, VA 22311

Phone: 800-DIABETES (800-342-2383)
Web site: www.diabetes.org

The American Diabetes Association is a good source of information on diabetes—definitions, risk factors, diagnoses, treatments, and living with diabetes (including materials on nutrition and exercise).

Children With Diabetes
Web site: www.childrenwithdiabetes.com

Children With Diabetes is an online resource for kids with diabetes and their parents, from a Q&A section to message boards and chat rooms.

Juvenile Diabetes Foundation International
120 Wall Street
New York, NY 10005
Phone: 800-JDF-CURE (800-533-2873) or
212-785-9500
Web site: www.jdrf.org

This resource provides news, research, and fact sheets on juvenile diabetes (also known as type 1 diabetes). Kids Online, an online resource especially for children, features news, fun, and important information.

DRUG ABUSE

See Alcohol and Drug Abuse, page 239

EMERGENCY PREPAREDNESS

Centers for Disease Control and Prevention (CDC)—Public Health Emergency Preparedness & Response
Public Inquiry c/o BPRP
Bioterrorism Preparedness and Response Planning
Mailstop C-18
1600 Clifton Road

NOTES

Atlanta, GA 30333
CDC Public Response Hotline:
Phone: 888-246-2675
888-246-2857 (Spanish)
866-874-2646 (TTY)
Web site: www.bt.cdc.gov

Through the CDC's Public Health Emergency Preparedness and Response, you can find information on specific agents and threats, preparedness and planning, and how to respond to emergencies.

Federal Emergency Management Agency (FEMA)
500 C Street
SW Washington, DC 20472
Phone: 800-480-2520 or 202-566-1600
Web site: www.fema.gov

The independent federal agency responsible for leading America's efforts to prepare for, prevent, respond to, and recover from disasters. At this Web site, you will find links to invaluable resources including:
•Ready.gov—provides detailed information on how to prepare for unexpected emergencies including potential terrorist attacks.
•Disasterhelp.gov—helps users find information and services for a wide variety of disaster situations.
•*Are You Ready? A Guide to Citizen Preparedness*, a book on how to prepare and respond to natural and man-made disasters. It is available online at www.fema.gov/areyouready or by telephone at 800-480-2520.

The US Department of Homeland Security
Washington, DC 20528
Phone: 800-BE-READY (800-237-3293) (for brochure)

TTY: 800-464-6161
Web site: www.ready.gov

This Web site will has tips for biological, chemical, and nuclear threats. It provides information on creating a family plan in the case of terrorist attack and on assembling a first aid kit. You may also download or call for a free brochure.

FIRE PREVENTION

National Fire Prevention Association (NFPA)
PO Box 9101
1 Batterymarch Park
Quincy, MA 02169
Phone: 617-770-3000 or
800-344-3555 (customer service)
Web site: www.nfpa.org

The NFPA provides a comprehensive range of fire safety information, including fire codes and standards, home fire escape planning, and seasonal fire tips. Sparky the Fire Dog (www.sparky.org) is a fun way for your child to learn about fire prevention.

Smokey Bear
Web site: www.smokeybear.com

Smokey Bear is a Web site for your child to find out about fire safety outdoors, including tips on proper campfire building and match safety.

FOOD SAFETY

Gateway to Government Food Safety Information
Web site: www.foodsafety.gov

This Web site is your complete online resource for accessing all government information on food safety, including materials from the FDA and USDA (see page 250).

Food and Drug Administration
Center for Food Safety and Applied Nutrition
5100 Paint Branch Parkway
College Park, MD 20740
Toll-free Food Info Line: 888-SAFEFOOD
(888-723-3366)
Web site: www.cfsan.fda.gov

By calling this infoline, you can find information on food safety and order related materials.

United States Department of Agriculture
Food Safety and Inspection Service
Washington, DC 20250
Phone: 202-720-2791
Meat and Poultry Hotline: 800-535-4555
800-256-7072 (TDD/TTY)
Web site: www.fsis.usda.gov

Use this hotline to report nonemergency complaints regarding meat, poultry, and egg products and to order food safety publications.

HEART DISEASE AND STROKE

American Heart Association (AHA)
National Center
7272 Greenville Avenue
Dallas, TX 75231
Customer Heart and Stroke Information:
800-AHA-USA1 (800-242-8721)
Stroke Information: 888-4-STROKE
  (888-478-7653)
Women's Health Information: 888-MY-HEART
(888-694-3278)
Web site: www.americanheart.org

The AHA is a good source of information on preventing and treating heart disease and stroke.

The Brain Attack Coalition
National Institute of Neurological Disorders and Stroke (NINDS)

Building 31, Room 8A-16
31 Center Drive, MSC 2540
Bethesda, MD 20892
Phone: 301-496-5751
Web site: www.stroke-site.org

The Brain Attack Coalition is a group of professional, voluntary, and government organizations whose mission is to reduce the occurrence of and disabilities and death associated with stroke. The Web site provides links to the patient information pages of the organizations involved and to the stroke information pages of many other institutions.

National Institute of Neurological Disorders and Stroke (NINDS)
Office of Communications and Public Liaison
PO Box 5801
Bethesda, MD 20824
Phone: 800-352-9424 or 301-496-5751
TTY: 301-468-5981
Web site: www.ninds.nih.gov

The NINDS, a part of the National Institutes of Health and the US Public Health Service, is the leading supporter of biomedical research on disorders of the brain and nervous system. Its Web site provides information on neurologic disorders and links to other neurologic resources.

HIV/AIDS & HEPATITIS
Division of HIV/AIDS Prevention
Centers for Disease Control and Prevention
National AIDS Hotline:
800-342-AIDS (800-342-2437)
800-344-7432 (Spanish)
800-243-7889 (TTY)
Web site: www.cdc.gov/hiv/dhap.htm

The National AIDS Hotline is a toll-free, 24-hour service that provides anonymous, confidential

NOTES

HIV/AIDS information and referrals. On its Web site, you will find fact sheets, FAQs, and other information including research and testing.

Hepatitis Foundation International
504 Blick Drive
Silver Spring, MD 20904
Phone: 800-891-0707
or 301-622-4200
Web site: www.hepfi.org

The Hepatitis Foundation International is a multi-lingual site that incorporates a newsletter and other information sources, events, links, and a kid's section. Information sheets on hepatitis can be ordered through the toll-free number.

American Liver Foundation
75 Maiden Lane, Suite 603
New York, NY 10038
Phone: 800-GO-LIVER (800-465-4837)
    or 212-668-1000
Web site: www.liverfoundation.org

The American Liver Foundation is a good source of information on hepatitis, research initiatives, and support groups for people with liver disease.

MEDICAL IDENTIFICATION BRACELETS

MedicAlert Foundation
2323 Colorado Avenue
Turlock, CA 95382
Phone: 888-633-4298
Web site: www.medicalert.org

MedicAlert is an emergency medical system that connects medical professionals with your vital records, 24 hours a day. Membership details are available on the Web site or by calling the toll-free number above.

MENTAL HEALTH

**Center for Mental Health Services
Knowledge Exchange Network (KEN)**
PO Box 42557
Washington, DC 20015
Phone: 800-789-CMHS (800-789-2647)
301-443-9006 (TDD)
Web site: www.mentalhealth.org

The Center for Mental Health Services is a service provided by the US Department of Health and Human Services. You can use the Web site or call to obtain consumer/survivor mental health information and fact sheets on a range of mental health topics, from schizophrenia to mood disorders.

National Mental Health Association (NMHA)
2001 North Beauregard Street, 12th Floor
Alexandria, VA 22314
Phone: 800-969-NMHA (800-969-6642)
800-433-5959 (TTY)
Web site: www.nmha.org

The NMHA provides a free infoline, referrals to mental health services and support programs in your area, and fact sheets on mental health for children and adults.

**National Mental Health Consumers' Self-Help
Clearinghouse**
1121 Chestnut Street, Suite 1207
Philadelphia, PA 19107
Phone: 800-553-4KEY (800-553-4539)
215-751-1810
Web site: www.mhselfhelp.org

This resource provides self-help information, referral services, advice on starting self-help groups, and technical assistance guides on issues such as fighting stigma and getting money for your self-help group.

NOTES

NOTES

PESTICIDES

Office of Pesticide Programs
United States Environmental Protection Agency
(EPA)
Web site: www.epa.gov/pesticides/factsheets/alpha_fs.htm

From this site, you can access "Citizen's Guide to Pest Control and Pesticide Safety" or you can order it from the National Center for Environmental Publications by calling 800-490-9198 or visiting its Web site: www.epa.gov/ncepihom/ordering.htm.

National Pesticide Information Center
Oregon State University
333 Weniger
Corvallis, OR 97331
Phone: 800-858-7378
Web site: www.npic.orst.edu

The National Pesticide Telecommunications Network is a toll-free telephone service (cosponsored by the EPA and Oregon University) that provides answers to your questions about pesticide-related subjects. It is staffed by pesticide specialists.

POISON CONTROL CENTERS

Check the front of the phone book for the number of a poison control center near you.

American Association of Poison Control Centers
3201 New Mexico Avenue, Suite 330
Washington, DC 20016
Phone: 202-362-7217
Web site: www.aapcc.org

This site does *not* provide information on specific treatments for poisoning, but it does let you locate your nearest poison control center.

POISONOUS PLANTS

Your local poison control center is a good source of information about poisonous plants. (Check the front of the phone book for a center near you.)

UCSD Healthcare
(affiliated with the University of California San Diego School of Medicine)
Phone: 800-926-UCSD (800-926-8273)
Web site: http://health.ucsd.edu/poison/plants.asp

This Web site has a listing of common poisonous plants, many with pictures.

RADON

**Consumer Federation of America Foundation
Radon FIX-IT Program**
Phone: 800-644-6999

The Consumer Federation of America Foundation, a nonprofit consumer organization, operates a free program for consumers whose homes are found to have elevated radon levels. The Fix-It Line, listed above, is in operation 24 hours a day, seven days a week.

US Environmental Protection Agency
National Radon Hotline: 800-SOS-RADON (800-767-7236)
Web site: www.epa.gov/iaq/contacts.html

The EPA provides information and publications on radon. Call the National Radon Hotline or contact your state radon office (details available at the EPA's Web site).

SENIORS

Seniors.gov
Web site: www.seniors.gov

An invaluable online resource that provides health and security information and services for senior citizens. This site facilitates immediate and convenient access to reliable health information, with an eldercare locator by state, as well as relevant federal agency and state Web links.

SPORTS INJURIES

American Academy of Neurology
1080 Montreal Avenue
St Paul, MN 55116
Phone: 800-879-1960 or 651-695-1940
Web site: www.aan.com

You can obtain the important guidelines for managing concussions in sports by contacting this organization or by visiting The National Guideline Clearinghouse at www.guideline.gov.

American Academy of Orthopaedic Surgeons
6300 North River Road
Rosemont, IL 60018
Phone: 800-346-AAOS (800-346-2267)
847-823-7186
Web site: www.aaos.org

Patient education brochures will tell you about the prevention and treatment of a range of sports injuries, including those related to specific sports.

National Youth Sports Safety Foundation (NYSSF)
1 Beacon Street, Suite 3333
Boston, MA 02108
Phone: 617-277-1171
Web site: www.nyssf.org

The National Youth Sports Safety Foundation (NYSSF) is a national nonprofit organization dedicated to reducing the number and severity of injuries youth sustain in sports and fitness activities.

Their Web site offers information on causes, treatment, and prevention of sports injuries in children.

STROKE

See Heart Disease and Stroke, page 250

TRAVEL

**Centers for Disease Control (CDC) and
  Prevention
National Center for Infectious Diseases
Traveler's Health**
1600 Clifton Road
Atlanta, GA 30333
Travelers Health Hotline Number: 877-FYI-TRIP (877-394-8747)
Web site: www.cdc.gov/travel

The CDC provides health information for international and domestic travel, including facts on vaccination, traveler's diarrhea, and disease outbreaks.

World Health Organization
Web site: www.who.int/ith/

This Web site has online information on medical kits for travelers, medical examination after traveling, travel advisories, healthy air travel, and vaccination requirements.

WATER AND BOATING

**American Red Cross
Public Inquiry Office**
2025 East Street NW
Washington, DC 20006
Phone: 202-303-4498
Web site: www.redcross.org

The American Red Cross offers swimming and diving courses, aquatic safety training, infant and preschool aquatic programs, and instruction on home pool safety.

US Coast Guard
Office of Boating Safety
2100 Second Street SW
Washington, DC 20593
Infoline: 800-368-5647
800-689-0816 (TTY)
Web site: www.uscgboating.org

Through this resource, you can find safety tips on all aspects of boating, as well as details on safe boating courses and a boating safety defect notification service.

WEATHER

American Red Cross
Disaster Safety Services
431 18th Street NW
Washington, DC 20006
Phone: 202-303-4498
Web site: www.redcross.org/services/disaster

The American Red Cross offers general tips on preparing for severe weather, as well as specific information on what to do in the event of earthquakes, floods, hurricanes, thunderstorms, tornadoes, and winter storms.

National Weather Service
1325 East West Highway
Silver Spring, MD 20910
Phone: 202-482-6090 (Public Affairs)
Web site: www.nws.noaa.gov

The National Weather Service Web site is a comprehensive online source of what's happening with the weather, including national and international weather conditions and maps. Through its Public Affairs department, you can find links to a wide range of severe weather and safety tips for floods, hurricanes, lightning, blizzards, tornadoes, and more conditions.

NOTES

INDEX

FAMILY MEDICAL RECORD

DATE OF BIRTH

Family Member   Date

_____
_____
_____
_____
_____
_____

MAJOR ILLNESSES OR MEDICAL CONDITIONS

Family Member   Date   Nature of Illness/Condition

_____
_____
_____
_____
_____
_____
_____
_____

SURGERY RECORD

Family Member   Date   Type of Surgery

_____
_____
_____
_____
_____
_____
_____

ALLERGIES

Family Member   Allergy   Usual Treatment

_____
_____
_____
_____
_____
_____
_____
_____

MEDICATIONS USED/DEVICES WORN (INCLUDING EYEGLASSES AND CONTACT LENSES)

Family Member   Medication/Device

_____
_____
_____
_____
_____
_____
_____
_____
_____

DATE OF LAST TETANUS BOOSTER

Family Member   Date

_____
_____
_____
_____

RECENT FOREIGN TRAVEL

Family Member   Date   Destination

_____
_____
_____
_____

LOCATION OF (FILL IN ALL THAT APPLY)

First Aid Kit _____

Asthma Medication _____

Anaphylactic Kit _____

Nearest Automated External Defibrillator (AED) _____

Any Other Special Equipment/Medications/Devices _____

_____
_____

FAMILY TELEPHONE NUMBERS

EMERGENCY SERVICES
EMS/Local Ambulance Service _911 or_ _____
Police Department _____
Fire Department _____
Local Poison Control Center _____
Local Hospital Emergency Room _____

MEDICAL/PHARMACY NUMBERS
Internist/Family Doctor _____
Pediatrician _____
Gynecologist _____
Dentist _____
Other Doctors _____
Local Pharmacy _____
24-Hour Pharmacy _____
Health Insurance/HMO _____
   Policy Number _____

HOUSE/AUTO NUMBERS
Electric Company _____
Gas Company _____
Homeowner's Insurance Company _____
Auto Insurance Company _____

FAMILY/FRIENDS
Mother at Work _____
Father at Work _____
Babysitter _____
Neighbor _____
Relative _____

YOUR HOME TELEPHONE NUMBER AND ADDRESS
_____
_____

NOTES

NOTES

NOTES

NOTES

NOTES

NOTES

NOTES